The Complete Cooking Techniques for the GAPS™ Diet

Monica Corrado, MA, CNC, CGP

selene river press
select books on nutrition health

Published 2019 in the United States by
Selene River Press, Inc.
PO Box 270091
Fort Collins, CO 80527
866-407-9323
info@seleneriverpress.com
www.seleneriverpress.com

Editor-in-Chief: Stephanie Selene Anderson
Editing by Heather Wilkinson
Book Design by Ellen Bryant
Photography on pp. 33, 49, 59–141, 161, 179, 181, 191, 199: Sandrine Perez. All rights reserved. Photography on pp. 145, 152, 163–175, 183, 187, 202–211: Lindsey Wohlman. All rights reserved. Monica's headshot on p. 221 by Erin Thames. All rights reserved.

Printed in the United States of America.
10 9 8 7 6 5 4 3 2 1

ISBN
978-1-943323-19-7 (Print)
978-1-943323-21-0 (PDF)
978-1-943323-22-7 (EPUB)
978-1-943323-46-3 (Mobi)

Note to the Reader: The ideas and suggestions contained in this book are not intended as a substitute for appropriate care by a licensed health care practitioner.

Contents

Introduction

When I began writing my original *Cooking Techniques* series, my goal was to introduce and explain the essential pillars of the GAPS diet, both in order of importance and in the chronology in which each book should be used in the GAPS healing protocol.

I launched the series with *Meat Stock and Bone Broth*. This book not only highlights the significance of Meat Stock but also explains the crucial differences between Meat Stock and Bone Broth. Meat Stock is the "healer and sealer" in the GAPS diet—it is used right from the beginning of the Intro. Bone Broth is not used until *after* the gut is healed, which means after the Intro or several months on Full GAPS.

In the second book, *Culturing Dairy*, the focus shifts to the role of cultured dairy in the GAPS diet. In addition to showcasing time-honored culturing techniques for cultured cream, soured (raw) cream, yogurt, kefir, butter, and ghee, this book also introduces the Dairy Introduction Protocol, a blueprint for how those with dairy allergies or sensitivities can successfully introduce cultured dairy products back into their diet.

Lacto-Fermentation, the third volume, is all about lacto-fermented foods and beverages: what they are, why you need them, and how to make them. Gut-healthy lacto-ferments are fundamental to rebuilding the gut flora. As Dr. Natasha Campbell-McBride notes in her foreword, the almost lost skill of lacto-ferments "is one of the reasons for the epidemic of abnormal gut flora in modern humans." Lacto-ferments are therefore required during the Intro of the GAPS healing protocol and throughout the Full GAPS diet as well.

I concluded the original series with *Seeds (Nuts, Seeds, Beans, and Grains)* to shed light on something that traditional cultures have known for centuries: how to unlock the immense nutritional power hidden in nuts and seeds by soaking, sprouting, and/or fermenting them. In addition to explaining the role of nuts, seeds, and beans in the GAPs diet, this book also includes a bonus chapter on how to introduce grains during the Transition diet.

Now, not only is all of this information gathered together, all in one place, but there is also a wealth of new material about GAP Syndrome and the individual stages of the GAPS healing protocol. It's all in the title: *The Complete Cooking Techniques for the GAPS Diet*.

Section I begins at the beginning: What exactly is Gut and Psychology (GAP) Syndrome? And why is it affecting the health of so many Americans, many of them children, with such a wide array of maladies?

By the end of Section II, readers will come to understand what elevates the GAPS diet to a *healing* protocol. These pages offer a breakdown of the GAPS diet itself: what it is, why it works, and how it promotes healing in four crucial ways.

The following three sections each venture into a different phase of the GAPS diet: the Intro diet, the Full GAPS diet, and the Transition diet. You will learn what foods to include, what foods to avoid, and what foods to slowly reintroduce over time.

Section VI fields questions about supplements on the GAPS diet—information that I am excited to present for the first time. Finally, included with all of this new material, I will answer a question I've often been asked: What should you eat after GAPS?

It has been a joy and a pleasure to bring you *The Complete Cooking Techniques for the GAPS Diet*. As ever, I wish you hope, health, happiness, and good food throughout your GAPS healing journey.

Section I | Why GAP Syndrome? Why Now?

Americans are sick. Brain function disorders are so rampant that our children suffer from a literal "alphabet soup" of maladies: attention deficit disorder (ADD), attention-deficit/hyperactivity disorder (ADHD), autism spectrum disorder (ASD), obsessive-compulsive disorder (OCD), and sensory processing disorder (SPD)—just to name a few.

Digestive system disorders have their own alphabet soup of names: irritable bowel syndrome (IBS), ulcerative colitis (UC), gastroesophageal reflux disease (GERD), small intestinal bacterial overgrowth (SIBO), and many more. To compound all of this, there is something else to consider: the new norm of food intolerances and sensitivities that so many people are experiencing these days.

Autoimmune disorders are also on the rise. Depending on who you quote, anywhere from eighty-five to a hundred or more autoimmune diseases affect untold numbers of Americans.

According to Dr. Natasha Campbell-McBride, many symptoms of these disorders stem from the same place: a damaged small intestine. In the Introduction for her groundbreaking book *Gut and Psychology Syndrome: Natural Treatment for Autism, Dyspraxia, ADD, Dyslexia, ADHD, Depression, and Schizophrenia*, Dr. Natasha writes:

> *Children with GAP Syndrome often fall into the gap—the gap of our medical knowledge…*
>
> *Apart from childhood learning disabilities: autism, ADHD/ADD, dyslexia, dyspraxia, and various learning and behavioral problems, there is another group of conditions which fit into the GAP Syndrome. These conditions are schizophrenia, depression, eating disorders, manic depression or bipolar disorder and obsessive-compulsive disorder.*

According to Dr. Natasha, though the symptoms may look different, they stem from the same place: a damaged duodenum, leading to malnutrition and all the havoc that malnutrition wreaks.

The role of a healthy digestive system is to both digest food—that is, break it down into usable parts—and also to absorb nutrients. If your digestive system is unhealthy or damaged, or if your diet includes refined and adulterated foods, some part of this process does not happen. Whether it cannot digest or cannot absorb, malnutrition will be the inevitable result.

To put it another way, GAP Syndrome is a *pathway to malnutrition*. Many people who go on the GAPS diet are suffering from malnourishment. The lining of their small intestine, where nutrients are absorbed, has been injured. This is an essential part of the digestive system, and the role of the GAPS diet is to provide the nutrients that are needed to slowly repair it. (The diet also rebalances the microbial landscape in the digestive tract, but more on that later.)

The duodenum is so important because it is the first section of the small intestine to receive chyme (partially digested food) from the stomach. Bile and pancreatic enzymes in the duodenum further breakdown fats and carbohydrates. Once the food is broken down, the small intestine absorbs the nutrients into the bloodstream, and the bloodstream then carries them to the liver for processing. From there, the nutrients are delivered through general circulation to the organs and tissues.

But for those with GAP Syndrome, this is not what happens.

In GAPS patients, the villi on the walls of the duodenum are damaged. The villi are small, hair-like structures that facilitate the passage of digestive fluids, keeping them in contact with food. Bad things happen when villi are damaged, including digestive fluids that run right through the intestine as if through a plastic pipe. The villi then flatten out and get thatch-like, clogging the absorptive capacity of the gastrointestinal wall.

When your body can no longer properly absorb nutrients, the consequences of malnutrition take over. It is as if you had not eaten any food at all. Except, that is, for partially digested food that feeds the pathogenic bacteria in your gut and, in some cases, releases toxins into your bloodstream. Even if most of these toxins never leave the intestines and are eliminated from the bowel, the bacteria can still trigger immune system reactions, brain dysfunction, and other problems. And if partially digested protein molecules enter your bloodstream, you may experience yet other food sensitivities and intolerances.

Why is all of this happening, and why is it happening now? The answer is simple: we have become accustomed to a steady diet of refined, processed, and chemically treated food that damages the digestive system. In children, such a diet can even prevent the digestive system from forming correctly in the first place. And without a healthy digestive system, malnutrition will result.

Healthy intestinal absorption works on the principle of "selective permeability." This means that some nutrients are allowed to pass from the intestines into the bloodstream, but harmful substances are not. Those with GAPS have increased intestinal permeability, or what is sometimes referred to as "leaky gut."

Qualified health professionals have long associated chronic malnutrition with all of the disease and brain function disorders I mention above: brain fog, ADD, ADHD, ASD, depression, dyslexia, dyspraxia, and schizophrenia, food intolerances and sensitivities, inflammation, and autoimmune disorders, to name a few.

Heal the small intestine, heal the symptoms. This is what the GAPS healing protocol is all about.

Section II | What Is the GAPS Diet? Why Does It Work?

First and foremost, the GAPS diet is a nutritional protocol. Because people with GAP Syndrome suffer from malnutrition, the GAPS diet focuses on highly nutrient-dense foods (plenty of protein, healthy fats, vitamins and minerals) that promote healing. Only when your small intestine can digest food *and* absorb nutrients will your body be properly nourished.

Why does the GAPS diet work? Gluten-free, casein-free, and dairy-free diets can remove irritants to the duodenum, but this alone does not guarantee or even encourage healing. To provide digestive and overall health, your diet must also provide nutrients for repair. The GAPS diet does both. It removes irritants *and* provides nutrients for repair, all while working to rebuild the microbiome, our gut flora.

But that is just scratching the surface. In the rest of this section, I will detail the four main ways that the GAPS diet promotes healing.

Step One | Remove Irritants and Stop Further Injury

You must stop irritating an injury if you want it to heal. The same is true of GAPS. The first step of this healing journey is to remove "offending" foods. These are foods that irritate or cause further injury. Your small intestine, due to its damaged state, cannot digest fibrous foods or foods with complex (large) molecules. Fibrous vegetables, for example, act like sandpaper on an open wound, which causes further injury to the duodenum.

Before we look at the following list of offending foods, please note that each individual is at a different stage of GAP Syndrome and a different stage of healing. Listen to your body. *If introducing any of these foods causes you digestive distress (bloating, cramping, diarrhea or constipation) or shows up undigested in your stools, it is a sign that your body is not yet ready to handle them.* Take a break from those foods for at least two weeks, and then try to introduce them again. Slow and steady is progress on the GAPS diet.

Here are some brief guidelines on foods that are not allowed because they can cause further injury. This information is not comprehensive, but I will come back to many of these foods later in the book.

Beans, legumes, and pulses

- *Intro*: All beans are excluded, with the exception of fermented white navy beans (for those who cannot tolerate nuts or seeds).
- *Full GAPS*: Most beans are excluded from Full GAPS, with the exception of lentils, white navy beans, green beans, and lima beans, all properly prepared.

Grains

- *Intro and Full GAPS*: No grains are allowed on the Intro or Full GAPS diet, whether they are gluten-rich or gluten-free. That means no corn, oats, rice, wild rice, barley, quinoa, amaranth, buckwheat, teff, wheat, spelt, khorasan (kamut), emmer, or einkorn. Name a grain, and it is not allowed until the Transition diet.

Soybeans

- *Intro, Full GAPS, and Transition*: No soy or soybeans, including soy sauce, tamari, tofu, tempeh, miso, and soy protein isolate.
- *Full GAPS*: Fermented natto may be included, as long as it is organic.

Fibrous vegetables

- *Intro*: No fibrous vegetables, including celery, celeriac (celery root), stalks of broccoli, stalks of cauliflower, Jerusalem artichokes (sunchokes).

Skin and seeds of vegetables, cooked and raw: The skin and seeds of vegetables can also irritate the gut. Listen to your body's signs and symptoms, one of which may be seeds or skins in the stool. If you see seeds or vegetable skins in your stool, it is a signal that you must peel your vegetables and remove their seeds. (Some individuals, especially those with ulcerative colitis, find it is best to peel and seed throughout the Intro.)

- *Stage 1 of Intro*: Your small intestine is delicate, and you must give it food that is soft and easy to digest, just like the first foods for baby. Peel and seed the following vegetables, then cook them until they are quite soft and mushy: carrots, beets, turnips, eggplant, zucchini, summer squash, winter squash, etc. You may also need to seed tomatoes, depending on the state of your healing.
- *Stage 4 of Intro*: Peel and seed raw vegetables, such as cucumbers, when you introduce them.

Fruit

- *Stage 6 of Intro*: Peel and seed all raw fruits, starting with apple.

Finally (though I hope it goes without saying), GMOs, chemicals, dyes, and preservatives are not allowed at any point on the GAPS diet.

> **No Plant GAPS.** Speaking of avoiding further injury, some people cannot tolerate plants in any form, not even cooked in Meat Stock and removed before eating. Thus, No Plant GAPS came about. Many people have been healed from severe cases of ulcerative colitis on No Plant GAPS—they eat only meat and Meat Stock, along with cultured dairy and good fats.

Step Two | Starve Pathogens

The second step to healing is to starve pathogenic bacteria. Pathogens thrive on sugar—all sugar, all carbohydrates. (There are only three kinds of macronutrients: fat, protein, and carbohydrate. If you are not eating fat or protein, you are eating a carbohydrate.) In order to starve the pathogens, you must remove all sugars from your diet for a while.

The definition of sugar is quite broad in the GAPS diet. It means sugar in all its forms, including fruit, starchy vegetables such as potatoes and sweet potatoes, grains, and most beans. (However, raw honey—a monosaccharide that the body does not have to breakdown—is allowed.)

In order to starve pathogenic bacteria, remove the following from your diet:

Starchy vegetables

- *Intro and Full GAPS:* Remove all starchy vegetables, such as potatoes (all of them), sweet potatoes, and cassava.

Sugar

- *Intro and Full GAPS*: Anything larger than a monosaccharide will feed pathogens and injure the gut. Sugar goes by many names, and you must remove them all: white sugar, turbinado sugar, cane sugar, barley malt sugar, beet sugar, brown sugar, corn syrup, corn syrup solids, date sugar, dehydrated cane juice, golden syrup, caro syrup, invert sugar, rapadura, sucanat, molasses, maple syrup, maple sugar, coconut sugar, maltose, galactose, sucrose, rice syrup, high fructose corn syrup, and lactose.

> **What about lactose?** The exclusion of lactose (milk sugar) is significant because it helps to define how long you will culture dairy in the GAPS diet. You will need to "culture long"—that is, for a longer period of time than is usual—to ensure that all of the lactose is predigested before you consume cultured dairy.

Starchy fillers

- *Intro and Full GAPS*: Examples of starchy fillers that are not allowed include guar gum, xanthan gum, locust bean gum, carob bean gum, and pectin.

Fruit

- *First four stages of Intro*: Exclude all fruit.
- *Stage 5 of Intro*: Introduce cooked, pureed apple. You may also add raw apple, pineapple, or mango to the therapeutic juice in this stage.
- *Stage 6 of Intro*: Introduce raw, peeled apple and other fruits.

However, keep in mind that some people never reintroduce fruit into their diet, particularly those who have had ulcerative colitis.

Step Three | Heal and Seal

Once you have removed all of the foods that can cause further injury, it is time to "heal and seal" the gut. This process requires two things: gelatin and amino acids, both of which are provided by Meat Stock.

When I teach about healing and sealing, I use the analogy of building a brick wall. The bricks are the amino acids—the building blocks of protein. The mortar (or sealant) between the bricks is the gelatin. You need both in order to heal and seal. And you get both from Meat Stock—it is *the* healer and sealer of the GAPS diet. Meat Stock is easy to digest, and it provides all the nutrients the body needs. As such, it is a fundamental part of the Intro.

But how much do you need? Stage 1 of the Intro is exclusively Meat Stock. You drink the stock, then you eat the meat and vegetables in the stock. You eat and drink it for breakfast, lunch, dinner, and in between for snacks. You will also use Meat Stock to prepare nourishing soups during this stage.

Stage 1 of the Intro is not a fast. Rather, it is meant to be deeply nourishing. As you progress through the Intro, you will consume less Meat Stock in each stage and steadily challenge your digestive system with foods that are harder to digest. This means foods with less liquid, such as stews and casseroles in Stage 2, and roasted meats beginning in Stage 4. However, you should still consume Meat Stock daily throughout all six stages of the Intro to be sure you are getting enough of the healing substance that is gelatin. (*Note*: For deep healing during the Intro, infants should consume one cup of Meat Stock per day, children three cups per day, and adults up to five cups per day.)

Even if you skip the Intro and start with the Full GAPS diet instead, Dr. Natasha suggests that you begin with Meat Stock exclusively to ensure that you are giving your intestine the nutrients it needs to heal. Do not begin with Bone Broth, which is allowed only *after* the gut has been healed and sealed, in most cases after you complete the Intro. This is important because Bone Broth contains high levels of glutamic acid, a substance known to aggravate the symptoms of an impaired nervous system.

Learn more in Section VII: Meat Stock and Bone Broth.

Step Four | Rebuild the Microbiome

The final step that elevates the GAPS diet into a healing protocol is the rebuilding of the microbiome in your gut. Once you starve out the pathogenic bacteria, the way is clear for repopulating your gut with beneficial bacteria. During the Intro, you accomplish this by consuming probiotics from lacto-fermented beverages, tonics, and foods, and also from cultured dairy products. (Probiotic supplements in pill form are usually reserved for the Full GAPS diet, or at least until Stage 3 of the Intro.)

Lacto-Ferments

You first add beneficial microbes to your diet in the form of what I call "ferment juice," which is simply the liquid of lacto-ferments. (Remember, starting with liquid is consistent with the goal of preventing further injury.) The juice from lacto-ferments—such as pickle juice, sauerkraut juice, or, better yet, a lacto-fermented tonic such as beet kvass—is your first source of beneficial lactobacilli. You add ferment juice right from the start of Stage 1 and slowly increase the amount as your body can tolerate.

In Stage 3, you add the lacto-fermented vegetables (that is, the sauerkraut/cabbage, not just the juice). By this stage your gut should be able to tolerate the partially digested cellulose of the vegetables. I say "should" because not everyone can tolerate lacto-fermented vegetables in Stage 3. Take heed of any clues, such as flatulence, bloating, or undigested food in your stool, that you are not ready to introduce them. Undigested food in the stool may also be an indication that the hydrochloric acid in your stomach is too low. If this is the case, increasing the amount of ferment juice you consume before each meal will help. (If it doesn't, you may want to add an HCl supplement, as explained in Section VI.)

Learn more in Section IX: Lacto-Fermentation.

Cultured Dairy

Whey from raw milk, yogurt, or kefir is another important part of the GAPS diet. Most people are not sensitive to whey, but even those who are find they can tolerate whey and/or cultured raw dairy. And still others can tolerate dairy, as long as it is from goats or sheep instead of cows. If you are concerned about introducing whey because of a past or known allergy or sensitivity to dairy, see the Skin Sensitivity Test (more on that later).

If you are not sensitivity to dairy, in Stage 1 of the Intro you may add whey and cultured dairy products, including cultured cream, soured (raw) cream, yogurt, kefir, butter, and ghee. If you are sensitive, slowly introduce as tolerated through all six stages of the Intro, until you can tolerate cultured dairy with ease at every meal.

If you could tolerate cultured *raw* dairy prior to starting the Intro, there is no need to begin with a small amount and then build up. Just continue eating the amount as usual. However, if you were eating *commercial* cultured dairy products prior to starting either the Intro or Full GAPS, you need to start at the beginning, with just a little bit, and work back up. Wait at least six weeks before you introduce cultured dairy products in order to allow your body to clear the commercial dairy from your system.

When you are able to eat large amounts—up to a ½ cup or more per meal—of as many varieties of lacto-ferments and cultured dairy products as you like, with no digestive upset, you will know that you are well on your way to a robust microbiome!

Learn more in Section VIII: Culturing Dairy.

Section III | The Intro Diet

The Intro diet is basically an elimination diet—a highly nutritious and delicious elimination diet. If implemented correctly, the Intro is not a starvation diet. The goal of the Intro is to eliminate offending foods while providing the body with all the nutrients, minerals, and enzymes it needs to rebuild.

What are offending foods on the Intro? As I mentioned in the previous section, offending foods do not promote healing on the Intro diet. In fact, they actively discourage healing in the following ways:

- They irritate the gut lining (for our purposes, the "gut" is specifically the duodenum of the small intestine).
- They break through the gut lining by entering the bloodstream as foreign proteins (because they have not been digested to the appropriate size).
- They kick off autoimmune symptoms (because they are foreign molecules in the bloodstream).
- They feed and encourage the growth of abnormal bacteria and yeasts (which give off toxins).

Should I begin the GAPS diet with the Intro? In most cases, yes. Dr. Natasha recommends beginning with the Intro because it is the most concentrated phase of healing and sealing. It is especially important as a starting point if you have any of the following serious digestive symptoms: reflux, diarrhea, abdominal pain, bloating, severe constipation, or swinging between constipation and diarrhea.

Why is the Intro diet important? What does it do? The Intro heals and seals the lining of the gut. Many disorders and dis-eases of the body and mind can be traced back to the health or dis-ease of the gut lining (that is, the lining of the small intestine). The resulting array of maladies, as I discussed at the beginning of the book, can include dyslexia, dyspraxia, depression, attention deficit/hyperactivity disorders, brain fog, autoimmune disorders, autism spectrum disorder, ulcerative colitis, schizophrenia, food intolerances, eczema, and seasonal allergies.

In order to clear these conditions and symptoms, we must *heal and seal* the gut lining. The Intro diet does this by:

- Nourishing the gut lining with the very building blocks that make it up: amino acids, gelatin, fats, vitamins, and minerals.
- Removing fiber and offending foods, such as gluten and casein, that would further inflame the gut lining.
- Providing probiotic bacteria that regenerate the cells in the gut lining.

What is the duration of the Intro? The time it takes to complete the Intro depends on the severity of your symptoms. Most people complete it in a matter of months. Some people can speed through it in few weeks. Others can take up to a year.

And some people never progress to the end and instead choose to remain at Stage 2, which provides complete nutrition for the body, indefinitely. This group includes adults with severe or long-term autism who will do best on Stage 2 for the rest of their lives.

What needs to be accomplished in each stage of the Intro? When you are on the Intro, you will follow three different tracks at the same time:

- **The diet** – The diet refers to the foods you eat at each stage of the Intro. Be sure to eat only the foods allowed on each stage. (See guidelines below. You may also refer to my GAPS Introduction Diet chart at the end of this section.)
- **Probiotic foods** – Probiotic foods include cultured dairy products (Section VIII) and lacto-fermented foods and beverages (Section IX). These are critical to the success of the GAPS diet as they provide beneficial bacteria (and yeast, in the case of kefir). They also provide soothing lactic acid, which feeds the intestinal flora and maintains a proper pH environment.
- **Supplements** – The food you eat on the GAPS diet is the primary and most important healer. However, Dr. Natasha also explains that certain supplements are critical to healing the gut. It is important to get the highest-quality supplements you can find—you do not want to add further toxins or cause stress on your body, brain, and digestive system with synthetic supplements. They must be pure, and they must not contain any ingredients that are excluded on the diet, so read the labels! Also bear in mind that you will not introduce vitamins and minerals until after your gut is healed and sealed—which means after the Intro. See Section VI to learn more.

How do I progress on the Intro? You will progress through the Intro diet in two ways: from within each stage, and from one stage to the next.

First, you progress within each stage by introducing foods in a specific order, testing them to be sure that your digestive system is ready for each one. As you will see later in this section, you introduce foods in the order they are presented in, from the top down. If you have a reaction (diarrhea, pain, bloating, or any other digestive discomfort) upon introducing a new food within a stage, do not continue with the food. Wait two weeks before you introduce the food again, and when you do, watch for symptoms. If clear, continue with the new food. If not clear, wait another two weeks or longer and try again. Do not rush!

As you progress within each stage of the Intro, you will also increase the amount of probiotic foods (lacto-ferments and cultured dairy) that you consume. Only after you have successfully introduced all of the foods within a stage do you go on to the next.

Second, you progress from one stage to the next. How do you know when it is time to go to the next stage? One of the gifts of the GAPS diet is that it requires you to listen to your body and get to know your symptoms. Symptoms of distress or dis-ease vary by person. The most typical symptoms are gas or flatulence, bloating, cramping, diarrhea, or constipation. Other symptoms include flare-ups of eczema or skin rashes, headache (including migraines), and exhaustion or fatigue. For those on the autism spectrum, symptoms may include increased acting out or withdrawal. It is essential to listen to your body for the unique-to-you way it expresses dis-ease or discomfort.

> **Bonus!** You can also use the Intro diet as a "reset" after a cold or flu, or upon returning home from travel. A few days on Stage 1 followed by a week or two on Stage 2 will have you back on track again.

Six Stages of the Intro Diet | An Overview

Remember, eat only the foods in each stage. Start each day with room-temperature water and a squeeze of lemon, as well as your probiotics.

If you suspect an allergy to a particular food (though one can only have a true "allergy" to protein), do a **Skin Sensitivity Test** before introducing it. (See the GAPS Introduction Diet Chart on page 18 for instructions.)

Stage 1 | Begin with the following:

Drink throughout the day:

- Homemade meat or fish stock prepared from joints, bones, meats, and bone marrow (can be made with chicken, turkey, beef, bison, lamb, pork, or fish).
- Ginger tea with a little raw honey.

Eat:

- Homemade soup made from homemade stock (may be blended or not).
- The meat, tendons, connective tissue, bone marrow, and vegetables from the stock.
- Use onions, carrots, broccoli, leeks, cauliflower, eggplant, squash, pumpkin, etc. Cook the vegetables in the soup very well, until soft like mush.
- Add 1–2 tablespoons chopped garlic just before serving.
- Do not use fibrous vegetables (celery, cabbage, broccoli stalks, cauliflower stalks).
- Do not use starchy vegetables (potatoes, sweet potatoes, celery root, Jerusalem artichokes, aka sunchokes).

Add probiotic foods:

- Add the juice of probiotic foods (dairy or vegetable based) to every bowl of soup.
- Start with 1–2 teaspoons a day (for 2–5 days), then 3–4 teaspoons a day (for another 2–5 days), until you can add a few teaspoons into every cup of Meat Stock and every bowl of soup. (Be sure the soup is not too hot, or the probiotics will be killed.)
- Dairy-based probiotics include homemade whey, yogurt, soured (raw) cream, cultured cream, and kefir. If dairy is not yet tolerated (by Skin Sensitivity Test or reaction), wait two weeks and try the Sensitivity Test again.
- Vegetable-based probiotics include sauerkraut, fermented vegetables, and vegetable medley (but for now, the ferment juice only), as well as beet kvass, fruit kvass, and cabbage tonic.

Stage 2 | Continue with all the foods from Stage 1 and introduce:

Raw, organic egg yolks:

- Add to soups and meat stock. (If you suspect an allergy, do a Skin Sensitivity Test first.)
- Start with 1 egg yolk per day and increase until you have an egg yolk in every bowl of soup and cup of stock.
- Dr. Natasha recommends up to 3 raw egg yolks per day for children and 6 per day for adults.

Stews and casseroles made with meats and vegetables:

- Do not use spices at this stage. Fresh herbs are okay.
- Be sure that every meal has a high fat content; add fat prior to eating.
- Add some probiotic foods to every serving, such as the juices from sauerkraut, fermented vegetables, or vegetable medley; or, if introduced, homemade whey, soured (raw) cream, cultured cream, yogurt, or kefir.

Fermented fish:

- Start with one piece per day and gradually increase.

Ghee:

- Preferably homemade, or the highest-quality store-bought ghee from organic, pasture-raised cows that you can find.
- Start with 1 teaspoon per day and gradually increase.

Increase in Stage 2:

- Daily amount of juices from sauerkraut, fermented vegetables, or vegetable medley; as well as beet kvass, fruit kvass, or cabbage tonic.

- If introduced, also increase daily amount of homemade whey, yogurt, soured (raw) cream, cultured cream, or kefir.

Stage 3 | Continue with all the foods from Stage 2 and introduce:

Avocado:

- Add 1–3 teaspoons of ripe, mashed avocado into every bowl of soup and gradually increase.
- If you think you are sensitive to avocado, do a Skin Sensitivity Test first.

Nut butter pancakes:

- Start with 1 per day and gradually increase.
- Make pancakes from organic nut butter, organic eggs, and cooked, mashed winter squash cooked in ghee, goose fat, duck fat, tallow, lard, or coconut oil (recipe on page 200).

Scrambled eggs:

- Scramble with ghee, goose fat, duck fat, tallow, lard, or coconut oil.
- Serve with avocado and vegetables (especially cooked onions) sautéed in a generous amount of fat.

Sauerkraut and fermented vegetables:

- At this point you will start eating the kraut or vegetables, not just the "juice."
- Start with a small amount and gradually increase to 1–4 teaspoons per meal.
- If there is any undigested food in your stools, wait 2 weeks before attempting to add fermented vegetables to your diet.

Increase in Stage 3:

- Fermented fish.
- Ghee and fats.
- Amount of juices from sauerkraut, fermented vegetables, or vegetable medley; as well as beet kvass, fruit kvass, or cabbage tonic.
- If introduced, also increase amount of homemade whey, yogurt, soured (raw) cream, cultured cream, or kefir.

Stage 4 | Continue with all the foods from Stage 3 and introduce:

Baked and roasted meats:

- Eat with well-cooked vegetables and fermented vegetables.

Cold-pressed olive oil:

- Start with a few drops and increase up to 1–2 tablespoons per meal.

Fresh carrot juice:

- Introduce on an empty stomach, either first thing in the morning or in the midafternoon.
- Dilute carrot juice with equal parts water.
- Start with a few spoons per day and gradually increase to 8 oz. per day.
- After a cup of carrot juice is well-tolerated, add celery, cabbage, lettuce, and fresh mint.

Baked goods made from nut flour or white navy bean flour:

- If nuts cause digestive disturbance, it is best to ferment the nut flour before baking.
- Use white beans if you cannot tolerate nuts.
- White navy beans must be soaked and fermented so you can easily digest them (learn more about white navy beans in Section X).

Stage 5 | Continue with all the foods from Stage 4 and introduce:

Cooked peeled apple:

- Add as apple puree, mashed with ghee or another animal fat (such as duck, lamb, tallow, lard, or goose fat).

Raw vegetables:

- Add lettuce and peeled cucumber first, then add carrots, tomatoes, onions, cabbage, etc.
- Do not add fibrous or starchy vegetables.

Raw apple, pineapple, or mango:

- Add to the carrot-celery-cabbage-lettuce-mint juice.
- Do not add citrus at this time.

Stage 6 | Continue with all the foods from Stage 5 and introduce:

Raw honey

Peeled raw fruits:

- Raw apple and other peeled fruits.

Some sweets allowed on Full GAPS:

- Baked cakes, muffins, or other sweet things made from nut or seed flour.
- Use dried fruit as the sweetener in baking.

How Much? General Guidelines During the Intro Diet

Probiotic foods (nondairy):

- Start with 1–4 teaspoons per meal and gradually increase to ½ cup per meal.

Probiotic foods (dairy):

- For whey, start with 1 teaspoon per day for 1–5 days and gradually increase to ½ cup per day.
- For homemade yogurt, soured (raw) cream, cultured cream (crème fraîche), or kefir, up to 1–2 cups per day.

Healthy fat:

- 1–4 tablespoons per meal of ghee, pasture butter, goose, chicken or duck fat, tallow or lard, extra virgin olive oil, coconut oil, or palm oil.

Egg yolks:

- 2–6 yolks per day (children).
- 4–8 yolks for per day (adults).

Gut and Psychology Syndrome (GAPS) Introduction Diet Chart

Stage 1

- **Homemade meat or fish stock with whey or ferment juice (probiotic juice) added to stock.** Ferment juice: start with 1 teaspoon in 1 cup and then in all cups. Gradually increase the amount of juice to 1 tablespoon per cup.
- *Note:* Prior to adding in whey, do a Sensitivity Test (see following). If clear, start with 1 teaspoon whey in 1 cup or bowl for 1–5 days, then increase to 2 teaspoons per cup for 1–5 days, until you are consuming 4–8 oz. of whey per day with meals. After whey is tolerated, add in homemade sour cream (cream cultured with yogurt culture), then homemade yogurt, then homemade kefir. *Note:* If a dairy allergy is suspected, do the Dairy Introduction Protocol (Section VIII).
- **Homemade vegetable soup made from meat or fish stock (well-cooked, nonfibrous vegetables).** Soup may be blended or not. Add probiotic juice (dairy or nondairy) to every bowl of soup—start with 1 teaspoon per bowl and increase. Eat the meat, cartilage, and marrow from the meat stock with each meal, as well as the fat from the stock.
- **Drink fresh ginger, mint, or chamomile tea between meals.**
- Move to next stage when all foods in this stage are well tolerated.

Stage 2

All of previous stage. Keep increasing the daily amount of homemade whey, sour cream, yogurt, or kefir. Keep increasing the amount of juice from fermented vegetables.

- **Add egg yolk to one bowl of soup** and continue until 2 egg yolks per bowl of soup for adults. When egg yolks are well tolerated, add whole, soft-boiled egg to soup bowls. *Note:* if you suspect an egg white allergy, do a Sensitivity Test first.
- **Add stews and casseroles made with meat and vegetables**, with probiotic juice added to each serving. Avoid spices. Fresh herbs and Celtic Sea Salt okay.
- **Introduce fermented fish or gravlax**, starting with one small piece per day and increasing.
- **Introduce ghee**. Start with 1 teaspoon per day and increase. *Note:* even if you are not introducing other dairy, introduce ghee.
- Move to next stage when all foods in this stage are well tolerated.

Stage 3

All of previous stage.

- **Add ripe avocado mashed into soups.** Start with 1–3 teaspoons per day and increase.
- **Add nut butter pancakes** made of organic nut butter, eggs, and squash. Fry in animal fat. Start with 1 per day and increase.
- **Add fried or scrambled eggs cooked in 4–5 tablespoons ghee or other animal fat**. Serve with sliced avocado and cooked vegetables. Cooked onions are especially good.
- **Introduce fermented vegetables**. Start with 1 teaspoon per meal and increase to 1–4 teaspoons per meal.
- Move to next stage when all foods in this stage are well tolerated.

Stage 4

All of previous stage.

- **Add meats cooked by roasting or baking.** Eat with cooked vegetables and fermented vegetables.
- **Add cold-pressed olive oil**. Start with a few drops per meal and increase to 2 tablespoons per meal.
- **Introduce fresh, clear carrot juice**. Dilute with water and add yogurt or sour cream/crème fraîche. Start with a small amount and increase to 1 cup per day. When carrot juice is well tolerated, add celery, cabbage, and fresh mint. Drink first thing in the morning or midafternoon on an empty stomach. Drink slowly—chew your juice!
- **Introduce baked bread made with ground almonds**, nuts or other seeds, eggs, squash, and fat. Start with 1 piece per day and increase.
- Move to next stage when all foods in this stage are well tolerated.

Stage 5

All of previous stage.

- **Add cooked, peeled apple** pureed with ghee or other healthy fat (duck, goose, lard, tallow, butter). Start with a few teaspoons per day and gradually increase. Add raw honey if desired.
- **Add raw vegetables**, starting with lettuce, peeled cucumber, carrot, and tomato (if not nightshade intolerant). Gradually increase. Watch for signs of intolerance (diarrhea).
- **Add apple, pineapple or mango**, or a combination to carrot/lettuce/mint juice. Avoid citrus at this time.
- Move to next stage when all foods in this stage are well tolerated.

Stage 6

All of previous stage.

- **Add peeled raw apple** and more raw honey. Gradually introduce raw, peeled fruits.
- Gradually introduce **more sweet things allowed on the diet**, using dried fruit for baked items.
- After digestive problems have cleared, move on to the Full GAPS diet.

Important Notes

Sensitivity Test: Prior to introducing any dairy, including whey, or any other food to which you suspect a sensitivity, do the Sensitivity Test. Place a small amount of the food on the inside of the wrist at bedtime. Upon waking, check the spot. If it is red and aggravated or itchy, wait another few weeks to introduce the food. Do another Sensitivity Test at that time. ***Do not attempt to introduce foods to which you have had an anaphylactic reaction!***

Meat Stock: Meat Stock is a meal. Eat the meat, drink the stock, and eat the vegetables. Meat Stock is cooked for a very short time (chicken 1½–2 hours and beef 4–6 hours) and has a lower amount of glutamic acid than Bone Broth. Only Meat Stock is eaten on the Intro diet.

How to know when to increase the amount of probiotic juice, ferments, or foods: The key to implementing the Intro diet is the word "gradual." Listen to your body. If you have abdominal pain, cramping or bloating, or stool changes, WAIT until the pain subsides and the stools normalize before proceeding.

Section IV | The Full GAPS Diet

When I'm asked about the Full GAPS diet, I explain that "Full GAPS" is like Paleo, with the addition of cultured dairy and lacto-ferments. On the Full GAPS diet, you will eat a variety of the best-quality ingredients you can find, prepared in your own kitchen, using traditional cooking methods. The Full GAPS diet includes meat, poultry, fish, eggs, vegetables, lacto-ferments, cultured dairy, saturated fats, and stock and broth, with some nuts and seeds thrown in.

Full GAPS is like French food without the bread and pastries, or Italian food without the bread and pasta. It is very much traditional "nose-to-tail" European fare with organ meats and the aforementioned ferments and cultured dairy products. The food our grandparents and great-grandparents ate. Food that served them well and kept them healthy.

Should I start with the Intro or skip to Full GAPS? Before you graduate to the Full GAPS diet, you must heal and seal your gut during the Intro. Ideally, this is the order they are meant to be completed: first the Intro, then Full GAPS. Even so, some people find it necessary to skip the Intro and start GAPS by way of the Full GAPS diet.

Dr. Natasha explains that you might want to start with Full GAPS if you fall into any of these categories: You have limited cooking experience; you are just starting to source pure food; or your career and/or extensive travel means you are not home enough to do the kind of cooking required on the Intro.

However, the most important thing is not where you start—it is just that you start somewhere! Your body is incredibly resilient, and you will benefit whether you start on the Intro or the Full diet.

Foods Not Allowed on the Full GAPS Diet

If it is not allowed on the Intro, it is not allowed on Full GAPS. I outlined many of the foods that are not "GAPS-legal" in Section II, but here is a brief overview:

Sugar

- No white sugar, maple sugar, coconut sugar, maple syrup, xylitol, or any sweetener that ends in "-ose" or "-ol" (exceptions include raw honey and stevia, if pure).
- No sugary drinks of any kind. You may have real sparkling mineral water with no added flavors or carbonation.

Processed foods

- No processed foods of any kind. (Yes, really!)

Beans

- No beans, including soybeans.
- Exceptions: lima beans, lentils, and white navy beans.

Grains

- No grains, sprouted or otherwise. This means no corn, wheat, triticale, spelt, rye, barley, amaranth, quinoa, teff, buckwheat, or oats.
- No products made from grains, such as flour, breads, bagels, rolls, crackers, tortillas, pasta, cakes, cookies, chips, popcorn, etc.

Starchy or fibrous vegetables

- No potatoes, sweet potatoes, cassava, Jerusalem artichokes (aka sunchokes).
- No celery, stalks of broccoli, stalks of cauliflower, etc.

Oils

- No processed oils.
- You may have extra-virgin olive oil (raw and unfiltered preferred), as well as palm, sesame, and coconut oils (preferably organic, cold or expeller pressed, and unrefined).

Foods Allowed on the Full GAPS Diet

All of the foods allowed on the Intro are also allowed on Full GAPS. Raw, cooked, and fermented vegetables are allowed. Fruit is allowed. All cooking methods are allowed, so you may roast, grill, bake, fry, and or sauté a wide variety of high-quality, nutrient-rich foods. You will eat the following foods every day on the Full GAPS diet:

Meat, poultry, fish, eggs

- Make sure to get the highest quality you can find.

Meat Stock

- 2–3 cups per day (see Section VII).

Vegetables

- Non-starchy and non-fibrous, cooked well and served with lots of good fat and salt.

Good fats

- Pasture butter, ghee, lard, beef, lamb, and bison tallow, duck or chicken fat.
- Extra-virgin olive oil, coconut oil, sesame oil, or palm oil.

Raw vegetables

- In moderation, with homemade salad dressings.

Cultured dairy

- Cultured cream, yogurt, soured (raw) cream, kefir (homemade and prepared from raw milk/cream preferred), yogurt cheese, hard cheeses, and raw milk if tolerated (see Section VIII).

Nuts and seeds

- All nuts and seeds, soaked, sprouted, or fermented and consumed in moderation (see Section X).

Section V | The Transition Diet (But Don't Jump Too Soon!)

Once you have been eating GAPS-style for a while—most likely for 2½ years or so—you will start to wonder if it is time to transition off the GAPS diet. Before you take this step, keep in mind that Dr. Natasha cautions that you do not jump too soon. Do not be *too* eager to start the Transition diet. After all, GAPS is a nutrient-rich diet that serves you, your digestive system, your immune function, and your brain function well.

Some people never go off of the GAPS diet because they just feel better on it—they have more energy and no symptoms. This includes people who remain at a particular stage of the Intro (usually Stage 2) because their symptoms will return if they move on.

How do you know when it is time to consider the Transition diet? As always, listen to your body. It will speak to you through symptoms that are unique to you, be they physical, emotional, or psychological.

You may be ready for the Transition diet if you have moved through all six stages of the Intro and completed a minimum of two years on the Full GAPS diet; if all of your digestive symptoms have been resolved; and if all of your other symptoms have been resolved.

When you are ready to transition, you will do it very much like you progressed through the Intro, by slowly adding new foods and looking for signs of digestive distress and/or the reoccurrence of any symptoms.

How do I introduce a new food during the transition? Start by preparing the new food as recommended. Eat one or two bites every day for a few days. If symptoms occur or recur, you are not ready to add that new food into your diet. Wait a minimum of two weeks before trying again. Once you successfully introduce the new food, eat it for a few weeks or more before introducing the next new food in the same manner. Proceed in this way until you have introduced all of the foods on the Transition diet. When none of these foods are not causing you any upset, you have officially transitioned!

What foods do I introduce in the Transition? Most of the foods that you will reintroduce are grains and starchy vegetables. They fall into three categories, which you will introduce in the following order:

Grains

- First buckwheat, then millet, and finally quinoa.
- *General guidelines*: You must prepare grains in a way that makes it easy for your body to digest them. You start by fermenting the grains prior to cooking. Later, once you have successfully introduced all of the other foods (including sourdough), you may use other traditional *Cooking Techniques*, such as soaking or sprouting. A final note on grains: be sure to serve them with plenty of good saturated fats when you eat them to modulate the sugar hit to your bloodstream.

Potatoes

- First new potatoes, then sweet potatoes, and finally other potatoes. (New potatoes and sweet potatoes both have a low glycemic index.)
- *General guidelines*: In order to counter the amount of starch (sugar) in potatoes, be sure to eat them with a very generous amount of fat. The best fats for potatoes are pasture butter, ghee, sour cream (soured raw cream), or cultured cream—or all of them at the same time. (Very therapeutic!)

Sourdough

- This means "soured dough." You will not add sourdough bread until later.
- *General guidelines*: The first sourdough you will introduce is sourdough pancakes made by soaking flour in homemade kefir. Again, start with just a bite of sourdough every day for a few days. If you have no reaction, you can gradually eat more of the pancakes.

After you have successfully introduced the sourdough pancakes, you may introduce other sourdough foods, including bread. However, this does not mean you should run out to the supermarket for a loaf of commercial sourdough bread any time soon. Most baked goods labeled "sourdough" from grocery stores or even bakeries may not be made from true sourdough. If you see vital wheat gluten or yeast listed in the ingredients, steer clear. Most of these products are not fermented long enough to predigest the gluten for you—which is what "sourdough-ing" is supposed to do. Ask for a traditional sourdough, made from a sourdough starter and proofed "long" (24 hours or more).

Note: See Working with Grains on the Transition Diet on page 211 for more information (including recipes and techniques) about introducing these foods.

Here is the complete list of foods to introduce on the Transition diet, in this order:

1. Fermented buckwheat
2. Fermented millet
3. Fermented quinoa
4. New potatoes
5. Sweet potatoes
6. Other potatoes
7. Sourdough pancakes
8. Buckwheat (soaked or sprouted)
9. Millet (soaked or sprouted)
10. Quinoa (soaked or sprouted)
11. Much later, grains with gluten

Section VI | Supplements on the GAPS Diet

"I cannot emphasize enough that an appropriate diet has to be the number one intervention in successful nutritional management of the GAPS child or adult" (Dr. Natasha Campbell-McBride, *Gut and Psychology Syndrome*).

Remember, the food you eat on GAPS is the primary and most important healer. But Dr. Natasha also explains that certain supplements are critical to healing the gut. It is important to get the highest-quality you can find—you do not want to add further toxins or cause stress on your body, brain, and digestive system with synthetic supplements. They must be pure, and they must not contain any ingredients that are excluded on the diet, so read the labels.

Dr. Natasha identifies a few supplements that are helpful on the GAPS nutritional protocol. The following "supplement" the nutrients on the diet itself:

- Therapeutic-strength probiotic
- Essential fatty acids
- Cod liver oil
- Digestive enzymes
- Vitamin and mineral supplements

You will find more details and the suggested dosages in *Gut and Psychology Syndrome*, but I will summarize the most important points here.

Therapeutic-Strength Probiotic

A therapeutic-grade probiotic is a good addition to the beneficial microbes you get from lacto-ferments and cultured dairy products on the GAPS diet. You can find many over-the-counter probiotics, but some are quite expensive.

As you navigate the options available to you, keep in mind that a good probiotic will have a *minimum* of twelve different species or strains of beneficial bacteria. The more the merrier. Look for a combination of lactobacilli, bifidobacteria, saccharomyces boulardii, bacillus subtilis (soil bacteria), and others. Dr. Natasha provides a wealth of information about each of these in *Gut and Psychology Syndrome*, under "Supplements for Children and Adults with GAP Syndrome." I encourage you to read it!

How much is a therapeutic dose? This simply means a large enough dose of the probiotic to have the effect that you are looking for. Remember, you want to win the war of populating your gut with beneficial microbes, and you will need enough new recruits to do it. Therefore, a therapeutic dose is a dose large enough to produce a die-off reaction. That means symptoms will get worse for a while before they stabilize. As with everything in the GAPS diet, start with a small dose and slowly work your way up.

Essential Fatty Acids

When it comes to omega-3 fatty acids, children and adults with GAPS need more EPA (eicosapentaenoic acid) than DHA (docosahexaenoic acid). You can get the essential fatty acids you need by including the following in your diet:

- **High-quality seed or nut oil blend**. Look for a ratio of two to one omega-3 and omega-6 fatty acids. Hemp oil and flax oil do *not* meet those requirements and are therefore not recommended.
- **Cod liver oil** (fermented or unfermented). Dr. Natasha recommends Green Pasture Fermented Cod Liver Oil (best with the high vitamin butter oil) and Rosita Cod Liver Oil. Though most people do well with the fermented cod liver oil, in my experience and that of many other GAPS practitioners, if you have a high histamine response—or if you cannot tolerate histamines at all—you may do best on unfermented cod liver oil. While cod liver oil provides some EPA and DHA, it is very high in vitamin A and D. Therefore, it is best to supplement with both cod liver oil and a good fish oil.
- **Fish oil**. Look for a fish oil with a higher ration of EPA to DHA. The best brand that I have found is Standard Process Tuna Omega-3 Oil and Calamari Omega-3 Liquid. (You will have to work with a practitioner to access them.)

General guidelines: Use high-quality brands, as oil extraction methods differ (cold extraction or pressed is best). Beware that the fragile oils may become rancid easily when not processed or stored correctly. Finally, it is important to purchase therapeutic-grade oils to prevent adding to the toxic load of the body.

Digestive Enzymes

Most children and adults with GAPS have low stomach acid, a condition known as hypochlorhydria. In some people, low stomach acid allows the overgrowth of pathogenic microbes and parasites. It is also responsible for nutritional deficiencies because it prevents the stomach from breaking down proteins. A physical sign of low stomach acid is undigested food in the stool. One of the first goals of the GAPS diet is to raise stomach acid by eating sauerkraut or drinking juice from sauerkraut prior to your meal. However, most people also benefit from betaine hydrochloride and pancreatic enzymes, usually for several months. See *Gut and Psychology Syndrome* for more details.

Vitamin and Mineral Supplementation

If at all possible, Dr. Natasha suggests that you do not introduce vitamins and minerals until after your gut is healed. Often, when the gut is healed and the microbes are back in business, you need much less supplementation. Also, many supplements can do more harm than good if they are not made of food. Synthetic vitamins cannot be used by the body anyway and only contribute to the toxic load of the liver. When you are ready to add vitamins or minerals to your protocol, keep the following in mind:

- Do not choose supplements that will aggravate the gut or contain ingredients that are not allowed on the diet. Liquid may be best.
- Choose supplements that will be absorbed rapidly.
- Keep supplements to a minimum. Let the nutrients of the diet do the healing for you.

Section VII | Meat Stock and Bone Broth

Originally published in a single volume under the title *Cooking Techniques for the Gut and Psychology Syndrome™ Diet, Part I: Meat Stock and Bone Broth.*

Foreword

> I would like to thank Monica Corrado for giving a clear clarification of the differences between meat stock and bone broth. In my book *Gut and Psychology Syndrome*, I include many recipes for meat stock. It's delicious to drink on its own and to make soup with. And the meat you use to prepare it can be made into a meal—just add a few cooked vegetables and a salad. I recommend that people start with meat stock. It's milder than bone broth and generally better tolerated by sensitive people. I prefer to use meat stock in the GAPS nutritional protocol rather than bone broth, particularly with children. When a good amount of healing has been achieved, you can start making bone broth if you wish. Thank you for doing this work, Monica!
>
> –Dr. Natasha Campbell-McBride

Meat Stock and Bone Broth

Introduction

It's amazing to me that the majority of people who go on the Gut and Psychology Syndrome (GAPS) diet created by Dr. Natasha Campbell-McBride miss the role of Meat Stock. They don't even know it's part of the GAPS diet, and they look at me in disbelief when I teach it in a GAPS cooking class or mention it in a talk. Yet Meat Stock is your saving grace in the kitchen, especially if you're implementing the diet for your family—or even if you just want to eat well and be well.

Even though Meat Stock is the cornerstone of the entire Intro diet, somehow readers skip right over the word "meat" and see only the word "stock." Many people familiar with traditional foods are well versed in how to prepare beef stock and chicken stock, especially from Sally Fallon's *Nourishing Traditions* and *Nourishing Broth*. But I imagine if they see only "stock" instead of "Meat Stock," they inevitably make Bone Broth instead. And this has proved to be a troubling misstep.

You may be wondering why I'm so strong about this point. It's because ever since *Gut and Psychology Syndrome* came out in 2004, hundreds, maybe even thousands, of moms and other caregivers have missed the critical first step of Meat Stock in the GAPS Intro diet. As a consequence, how many children with nervous system disorders have endured aggravated symptoms—including seizures, stimming, and nervous tics—by skipping this pillar of the Intro diet? Everyone needs to heal and seal their guts with Meat Stock before moving on to Bone Broth, but especially children with ADD, ADHD, and autism spectrum disorder.

In this section, you'll gain a clear understanding of the difference in the application of and results from these very important foods: Meat Stock and Bone Broth.

Meat Stock = GAPS Intro Diet
Bone Broth = GAPS Full Diet

What is Meat Stock? And what is Bone Broth for that matter? Aren't they the same? In a word, no, they are not. For the purposes of the GAPS diet, you use Meat Stock exclusively during the Intro diet. You don't use Bone Broth until your gut is healed and sealed and you're ready to start on the Full GAPS diet.

Why the Introduction Diet, aka "The Intro"?

Heal and seal the gut! So many disorders and diseases of the body and mind can be traced back to the health or disease of the gut lining (that is, the lining of the small intestine). The Intro diet, or just "Intro," is basically an elimination diet, but a highly nutritious and delicious elimination diet. It's nutrient dense, providing the body with all the nutrients, minerals, and enzymes it needs to detox and rebuild. The Intro is composed of six stages. Each stage introduces new foods back into the diet, including ferments, fats, and dairy. For an easy-to-follow and detailed chart, see the GAPS Introduction Diet Chart in Section III.

One more time with feeling: I wrote *Meat Stock and Bone Broth* to aid those who are implementing the Gut and Psychology Syndrome healing protocol. This isn't a culinary class. Rather than define stock or broth in culinary terms, I define them with regard to this diet only. This knowledge may not be transferrable outside of the protocol.

Meat Stock and Bone Broth

Understanding the Purpose of Meat Stock and Bone Broth

1

One of the things that intimidates many people when starting the GAPS diet, or even contemplating it, is the amount of stock required on the Intro. But once you know more about Meat Stock, you'll see there's no need to worry!

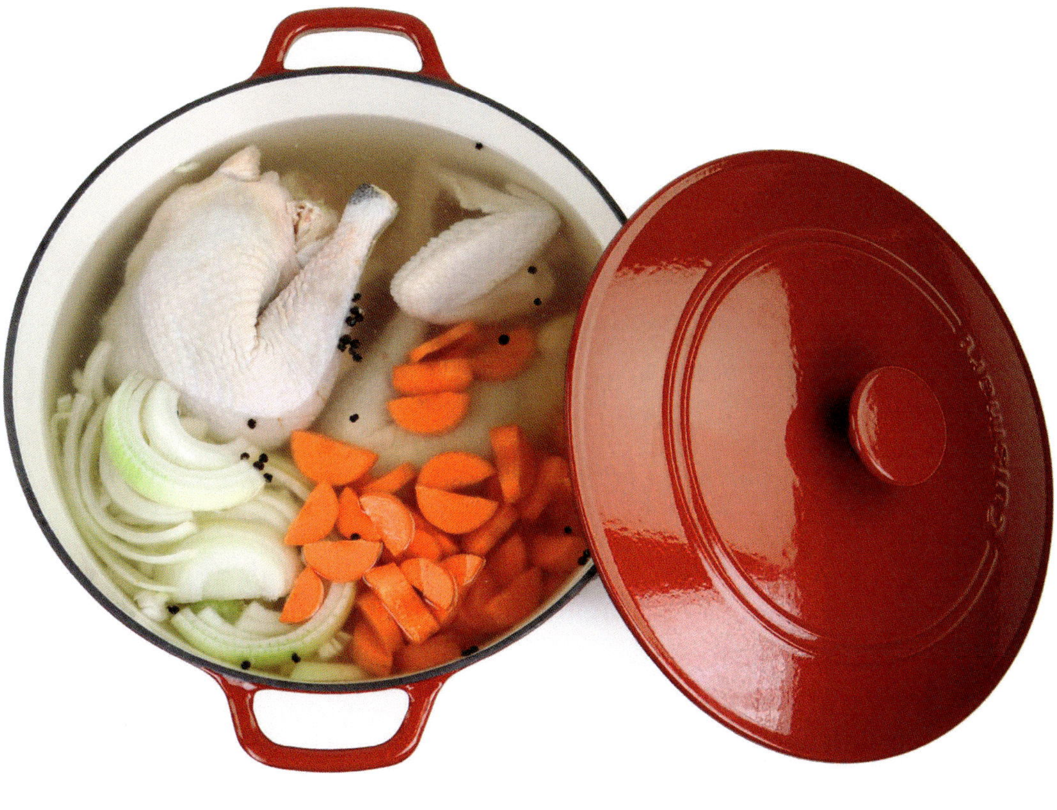

Meat Stock: When and Why

When you think of the Intro diet, Meat Stock is the first thing that should come to mind. It's the only stock used during the Intro of the GAPS diet. Period.

Intro Diet = Meat Stock

There are very good reasons that Meat Stock, and only Meat Stock, is used during the six stages of the Intro diet:

- The gelatin and amino acids in Meat Stock heal the gut lining, aka the lining of the small intestine—specifically, the duodenum.
- Meat Stock is low in glutamic acid. This is important because people sensitive to MSG may experience nervous system symptoms from high levels of glutamic acid and free glutamates if the gut is not yet healed.
- Meat Stock heals the gut, allowing one to advance to the full diet and further healing.

Symptoms of Sensitivity to MSG

- Headache and migraines
- Mild chest pain
- Flushing
- Numbness or burning, especially in and around the mouth
- Facial pressure or swelling
- Sweating
- Asthma, shortness of breath
- Hives
- Swelling of the face, mouth, and tongue
- Rhinitis or post-nasal drip
- Tendonitis and joint pain
- Flu-like symptoms
- Anxiety or panic attacks
- Hyperactivity in children
- Nervous system disorders
- Difficulty focusing

These are just to name a few; there are many more symptoms of MSG sensitivity.

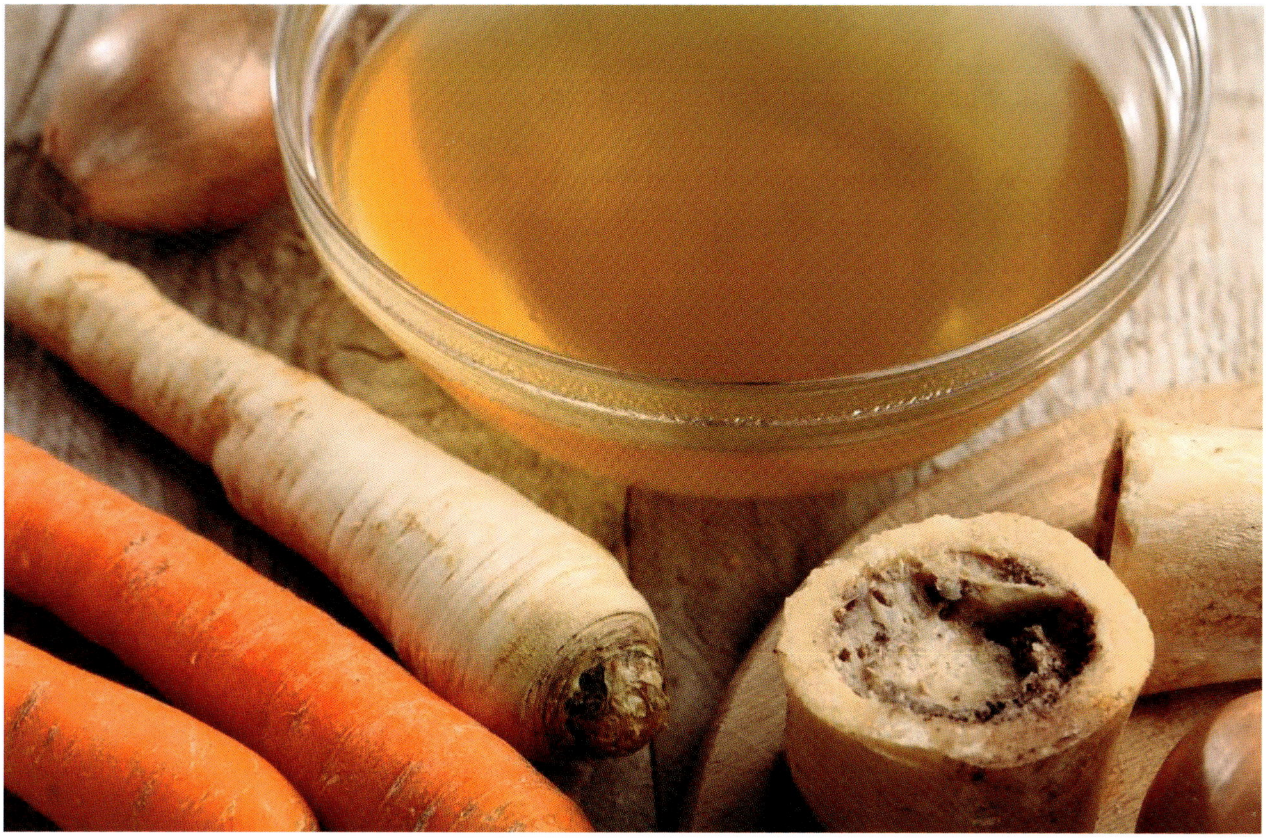

Bone Broth: When and Why

When you think of the full diet, Bone Broth is the first thing that should come to mind. You use it only after the gut is healed and sealed—that is, **after** you graduate from the Intro and advance to the Full GAPS diet.

Full Diet = Bone Broth

Bone Broth is very high in glutamic acid, which can trigger nervous system symptoms if the gut is not yet healed. That's what the Intro diet is for: healing the gut lining. Once your gut is healed, you may consume Bone Broth.

Warning signs that you've moved too quickly from Meat Stock to Bone Broth may include die-off reactions such as rashes or skin eruptions, eczema, diarrhea, vomiting, nausea, constipation, or nervous system dysfunction in those prone to seizures. (Bone Broth may trigger seizures in those who are prone to them.) For those with ADD, ADHD, Autism Spectrum Disorders, or MS, nervous system agitation can be a warning sign.

The high concentration of glutamic acid in Bone Broth can trigger these symptoms if you still have a leaky gut or leaky membranes in the brain. In fact, the presence of the symptoms means that the gut is still porous and further healing is needed.

Symptoms of a Leaky Gut

- Bloating, gas, cramps, loose stools, aches and pains
- IBS, Crohn's disease, ulcerative colitis
- Candida overgrowth or small intestinal bacterial overgrowth (SIBO)
- Food sensitivities
- Seasonal allergies
- Autoimmune disease or condition
- Chronic fatigue or tired all the time
- Fibromyalgia
- Thyroid issues
- Malabsorption
- Eczema, acne, psoriasis, and other chronic skin issues
- Mood issues, including depression, anxiety, and mood swings
- Autism
- Other brain function disorders, including difficulty with focus and memory, ADD, ADHD, and Asperger's
- Difficulty losing weight
- Achy or swollen joints, sensitivity to free glutamates, including MSG, glutamine, and glutamic acid
- Other inflammatory conditions

So why bother with Bone Broth at all?

- Bone Broth comes with all the benefits of Meat Stock. Once your gut is healed and sealed, it's a healthful addition to your diet and your cooking repertoire. See Chapter 3: Bone Broth—It's All About the Bones.
- Bone Broth is sustainable: you make it from the bones from your Meat Stock, gleaning the last goodness from them—especially a high concentration of easily absorbed minerals and nutrients made available by long, slow cooking at low temperatures.

Meat Stock vs. Bone Broth: Telling Them Apart

Meat Stock is the stock derived from cooking a piece or pieces of meat with a joint for a relatively short amount of time. Some examples are turkey legs or thighs, a whole chicken cut up, beef or lamb shank, beef soup bones, or turkey or lamb neck bones. We're talking a lot of meat to little bone. Meat Stock is cooked for a relatively short amount of time, about 1½–3 hours for poultry and no more than 6 hours for beef, bison, or lamb. These times are a bit longer in a slow cooker.

Making meat stock is making a meal. You eat the meat, cartilage, tendons or connective tissue, and vegetables, and you drink the stock. You consume everything but the bones, which you may save to make Bone Broth. (More on that later.) On the Intro diet, you consume Meat Stock at every meal and throughout your day.

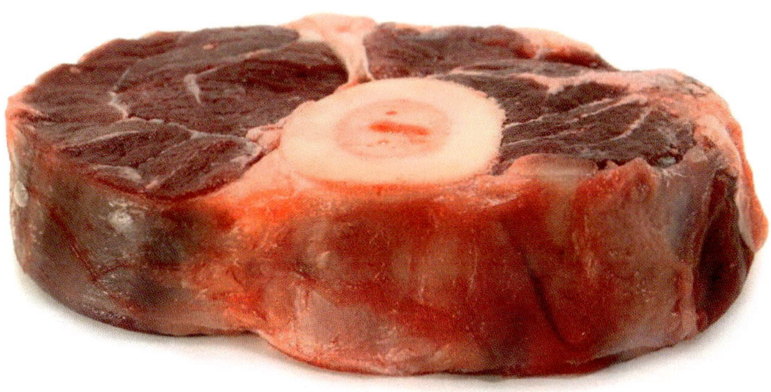

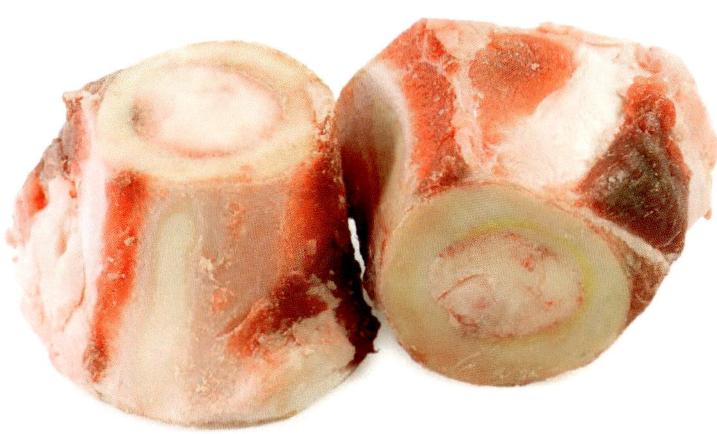

Meat Stock = A Meal
Bone Broth = Broth

Bone Broth is the broth derived from cooking a lot of bones for a long period of time. The purpose is to prepare a large quantity of broth at one time. On the full diet, you use it as a beverage throughout the day, and you can use it as the foundation of vegetable soups and stews.

Meat Stock is a lot of meat with a few bones, cooked for a short period of time.

Bone Broth is a lot of bones with a little meat, cooked for a long period of time.

Bone Broth and Meat Stock at a Glance

This simple chart below sums up the differences in bone ratio and cook time of Bone Broth and Meat Stock, as well as showing what to consume and what to discard.

	Bone Broth	Meat Stock
Bone Ratio	Approximately 80 percent boney bones (marrow bones, knuckles, joints, neck) to 20 percent meaty bones (ribs)	Approximately 20 percent boney bones to 80 percent meaty bones. (This ratio is often accomplished with the meaty bone itself as you don't need to add in additional boney bones. More details below.)
Cook Time	Simmered for a long period of time: 6–24 hours for chicken; 24–72 hours for beef Suggested times for slow cooker: 48 or more hours on low for beef or bison; 24 hours on low or 8–10 hours on high for chicken **Note:** you'll need to halve your recipe for beef Bone Broth as it will not fit in a slow cooker.	*Cooked in a low oven at about 300°F or on the burner, covered:* 1½–3 hours for chicken or other poultry; 3–6 hours for beef, bison, or lamb. *Cooked in a slow cooker set to low:* 6 hours for chicken; start with 2 hours on high and then 8 hours on low for beef, bison, or lamb.
Consume	Broth only. Discard meat, bones, and vegetables after making now that all of their goodness is in the broth!	Meat, cartilage, connective tissue, tendons, and vegetables. Reserve the bones for use in Bone Broth when on the Full GAPS diet.

A note on slow cookers: While you cook Meat Stock for a shorter period of time than Bone Broth, it will take longer in a slow cooker. Most take a long time to come to temperature, which means an extended cooking time. If your slow cooker can bring the Meat Stock to temperature as quickly as your stove, then use the stovetop cooking time. Learn more about slow cookers in Chapter 4: Everything Else You Need to Know.

Meat Stock and Bone Broth: The Benefits of Each

Meat Stock and Bone Broth both contain the super-nutrient gelatin, making them high in hydrophilic colloids that attract digestive juices and therefore aid in digestion. (Hydrophilic means to attract water.)

Gelatin also improves the integrity of collagen. This is apparent in the improved appearance of the skin and in decreased inflammation of the digestive tract.

Gelatin has also been known to enhance healing of many digestive and other disorders, including anemia, diabetes, colitis, rheumatoid arthritis, and even cancer.

Both Meat Stock and Bone Broth act as a "protein-sparer." That means when you consume stock or broth with a meal, you utilize the protein you consume more efficiently, which will then reduce the amount you need to eat.

Both Meat Stock and Bone Broth promote the secretion of hydrochloric acid (HCl) in the stomach, where it's needed to break down proteins. Insufficient HCl can lead to a whole host of symptoms, including acid reflux, skin disorders, anemia, osteoporosis, rheumatoid arthritis, vitiligo, asthma, alkalinity, food allergies, and more. What's more, most Americans have insufficient HCl.

Because it's cooked longer, Bone Broth is higher in electrolytic minerals. These are in an electrolytic state, so as they're drawn out of the bones and into the broth, they're easily absorbed by the body. (Think rehydration also—electrolytic mineral-rich Bone Broth is a natural rehydration drink, like coconut water.)

Bone Broth is also higher in proline and glycine, the same amino acids (with the exception of histidine) found in Meat Stock. These amino acids help to heal and strengthen connective tissue.

For more information about the healing properties of gelatin, Bone Broth, and HCl, see the Resources section at the end of this book. The following chart will also help you better understand some of the important nutritional components of Meat Stock and Bone Broth.

Comparative Analysis of Amino Acids in Short Cooked Chicken Meat Stock and Long Cooked Chicken Bone Broth (serving size 8 fl. oz.)

Amino Acids	Meat Stock (short cooked)	Bone Broth (long cooked)
Aspartic Acid	161 mg	553.33 mg
Threonine	70.33 mg	214 mg
Serine	85.67 mg	242.67 mg
Glutamic Acid	366.67 mg	1,013.33 mg
Proline	242.33 mg	986.67 mg
Glycine	450 mg	1,773.33 mg
Alanine	214.33 mg	773.33 mg
Valine	63.67 mg	181 mg
Isoleucine	43 mg	131.67 mg
Leucine	92.33 mg	276.33 mg
Tyrosine	34 mg	76.33 mg
Phenylalanine	56.67 mg	192.33 mg
Lysine	127.67 mg	303 mg
Histidine	98.67 mg	93.67 mg
Arginine	170.67 mg	696.67 mg
Cystine	<23.77 mg	<24.03 mg
Methionine	26.13 mg	96.33 mg

Lab analysis performed by Covance Laboratories, Madison, Wisconsin. For the sake of comparison, both formulas used organically raised chickens from Mary's. Kim Schuette had the Bone Broth analyzed for lead and levels were found to be <1.67 ppb, well within acceptable levels.

Great thanks to Kim Schuette of Biodynamic Wellness for the use of the chart and lab analysis.

Meat Stock and Bone Broth

More on Meat Stock—It's a Meal!

2

One of the most significant qualities of Meat Stock is that it's a meal! You eat the meat and the vegetables and drink the stock. You can make Meat Stock with any piece of meat or poultry that has a bone with a joint or connective tissue in it. The following chart sums up the ingredients you'll need to start making your own Meat Stock, followed by specific recipes.

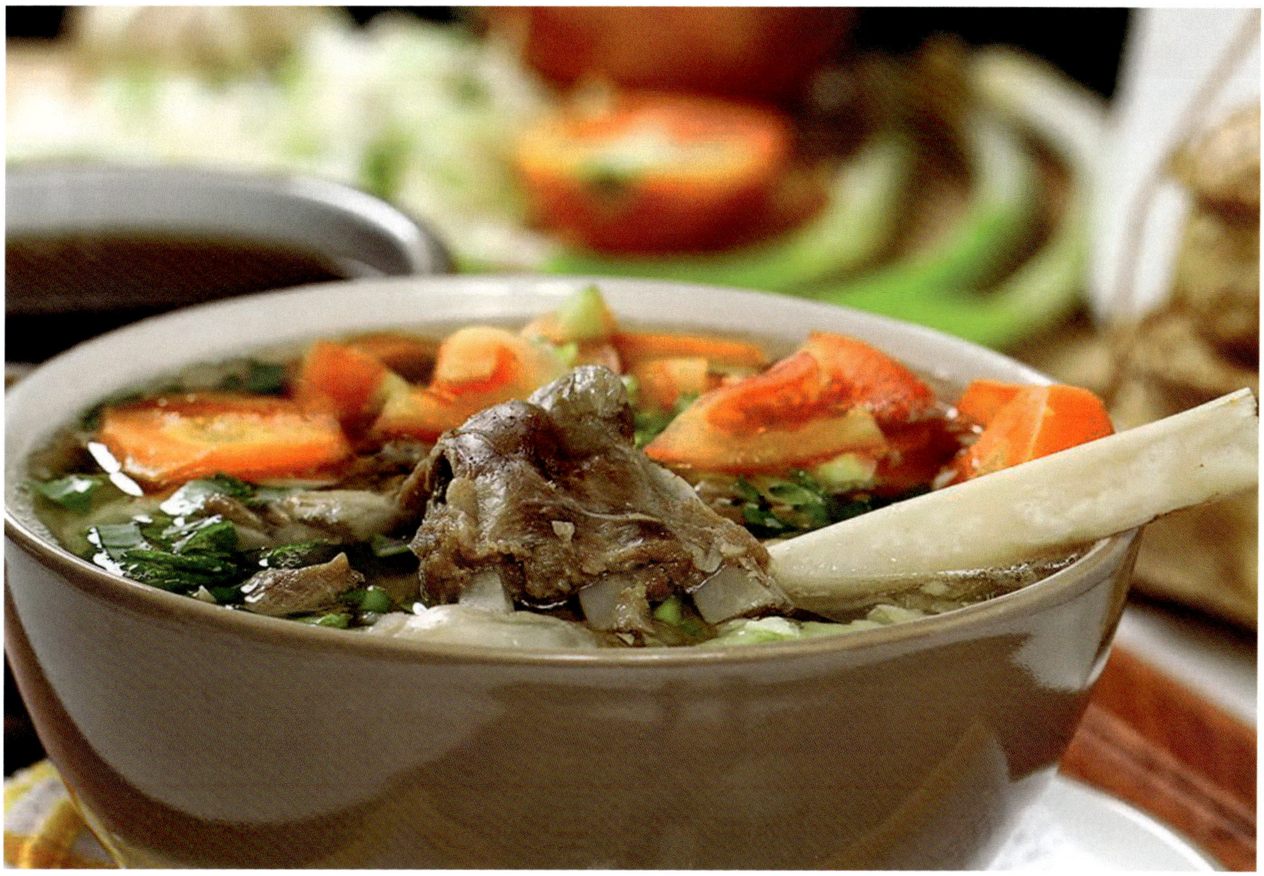

Handy Meat Stock Chart

Protein	Chicken, Goose, or Duck	Turkey	Beef, Lamb, Pork, Bison, or Game	Fish
Amount	Whole or half bird Giblets or 3–4 lbs. necks, backs, or wings (or a combination)	About 2–3 lbs. thighs or legs (or a combination) Giblets or necks, backs, and wings	About 2–3 lbs. meaty joints, bones, or marrow bones Meaty soup bones or soup bones Shanks, meaty ribs, or marrow bones with a piece of meat on the bone	About 3 lbs. bones, fins, skins, and head
Vegetables (optional)	Carrots, onions, zucchini, all non-starchy, and nonfibrous vegetables			
Water	3–4 quarts to cover by 1–2 inches. The amount of water is determined by the amount of meat in the Dutch oven and the size of the Dutch oven itself.			
Spices	1 teaspoon black peppercorns and good quality sea salt to taste			
Type of pot	5–6 quart Dutch oven, covered (preferred, but slow cooker okay)			
Time	**Stove or oven:** 1½ –3 hours simmered on the stove or cooked in 300°F oven, covered **Slow cooker:** 1 hour on high, then 6 hours on low	**Stove or oven:** 2½ –3½ hours simmered on stove or cooked in 300°F oven, covered **Slow cooker:** 1 hour on high, then 8 hours on low in a slow cooker	**Stove or oven:** 3–6 hours simmered on stove or cooked in 300°F oven, covered **Slow cooker:** 2 hours on high, then 8 hours on low *For lamb:* 2 hours on high, then 6 hours on low	**Stove or oven:** 1–1½ hours simmered on stove or cooked in 300°F oven, covered **Slow cooker:** 1 hour on high, then 1 hour on low
What to eat from Meat Stock	Eat meat, tendons, and fat, and the vegetables if you used them (all of which are discarded for Bone Broth)			

Please note that vinegar is **not** used in Meat Stock. See Chapter 3: Bone Broth—It's All About the Bones for more details.

Meat Stock Recipes

The following recipes may be used throughout the entire GAPS diet. Meat Stock is specific to the Intro diet, but you may eat it throughout the full diet and after graduating from GAPS. Each recipe corresponds to one or more of the six stages of the Intro or Full GAPS diet, as noted below.

Before we go on to the recipes, I just want to highlight:

> **No fibrous vegetables, please!** You may notice that celery is absent from the Meat Stock recipes. This is for good reason—the Intro diet doesn't allow any fibrous vegetables, and celery is a known culprit! During the Intro, avoid all varieties of cabbage and celery, plus the stalks and any other fibrous parts of broccoli and cauliflower. Also remove the skin and seeds from all squash.

Meaty Bones vs. Boney Bones

What is a "meaty bone"? Meaty bones are mostly meat, with a little bone or joint and some connective tissue around it. For beef, lamb or pork they can be meaty soup bones, shanks, hocks, meaty neck bones, and short ribs. For chicken or poultry they can be whole legs or thighs or a whole bird cut up. **Hint:** Meat Stock is made from meaty bones.

What is a "boney bone"? Boney bones have little or no meat on them, and they're used to make Bone Broth. For beef, lamb, or pork Bone Broth they include marrow bones (aka long bones) and joints such as knuckles, necks, and spines. For chicken or poultry they can be long bones (leg and thigh), or wings, necks, and backs.

Basic Meat Stock: Turkey or Chicken

When you're on the Full GAPS diet, you may wish to brown the meat in lard, tallow, ghee, or another healthy fat as a first step in making Meat Stock. Serves 4.

Ingredients

2–3 lbs. pastured skin-on turkey or chicken (thighs or quarters) or a whole pastured chicken, cut up
3–4 carrots, coarsely chopped
1 small onion, peeled and quartered
Handful black peppercorns
1–2 teaspoons Celtic Sea Salt
2–3 sprigs fresh rosemary or thyme
Water to cover by 2 inches
Garlic cloves, to finish

Instructions

1. Place all ingredients in 5–6 quart Dutch oven. Bring to a boil. Skim and discard the scum.
2. Keep at a low simmer for 1½–3 hours, or place pot in the oven and cook at 300°F for 3 hours. If using slow cooker, cook for 1 hour on high, then 6 hours on low.

Stage 1 of Intro: Serve meat and vegetables with a cup of stock alongside. Using a garlic press, add a small clove to each cup. Add some good sea salt or whey. Or add probiotic juice from vegetable ferments or cultured dairy products like homemade crème fraîche or yogurt (unless there's a dairy sensitivity). Eat all connective tissues such as cartilage and tendons from meat and joints.

Stage 2 of Intro: Add raw egg yolks to each cup of Meat Stock you drink, starting with 1 per day and working up to several per day.

Basic Meat Stock: Beef, Bison, or Lamb

When you're on the Full GAPS diet, you brown the meat in lard, tallow, ghee, or another healthy fat as the first step in making Meat Stock. Serves about 4.

Ingredients

2–3 lbs. grass-fed beef, bison, or lamb shanks
3–4 carrots, coarsely chopped
1 small onion, peeled and quartered
Handful black peppercorns
1–2 teaspoons Celtic Sea Salt
2–3 sprigs fresh rosemary or thyme
Water to cover by 2 inches
2–3 garlic cloves, to finish

Instructions

1. Place all ingredients in a 5–6 quart Dutch oven. Bring to a boil. Skim and discard any scum.

2. Leave on the stove at a low simmer for about 3–6 hours or place pot in the oven and cook at 300°F for 3 hours. If using slow cooker, cook beef or bison on high for 2 hours, then on low for 8–10 hours. Lamb will need about 6 hours on low, after bringing up the temperature for 2 hours on high.

Stage 1 of Intro: Serve meat and vegetables with a cup of Meat Stock. Using a garlic press, add a small clove to each cup, along with some good sea salt or whey. Or use probiotic juice from vegetable ferments or cultured dairy products like homemade crème fraîche or yogurt (unless there's a dairy sensitivity). Eat all connective tissues such as cartilage and tendons from meat and joints.

Stage 2 of Intro: Add raw egg yolks to each cup of Meat Stock you drink, starting with 1 per day and working up to several per day.

Why We Love Meat Stock Leftovers! Six Variations on a Theme

The beauty of Meat Stock is that once you make your stock, you get a meal to boot. And then you can do wonders with the leftovers too. This is truly an efficient way to feed you and yours. Here are some ideas for tasty leftovers:

Just reheat what you've made and eat the same meal again. Yum—super easy!

Stage 2 of Intro: Pick the meat off the bones. Freeze the bones to make Bone Broth later. Place the meat back into the pot—now you have stew. You may need to add a few more cooked vegetables, depending on how many you ate the first time.

Stage 2 of Intro: Pick the meat off the bones, reserve. Strain out any cooked vegetables, reserve. Bring the Meat Stock to a boil, then skim and discard any scum. Add freshly chopped vegetables. Reduce temperature and simmer about 20 minutes, or until vegetables are cooked. Add the meat and any reserved vegetables to the pot. Voila! Another pot of hearty stew.

Stage 1+ of Intro: Take the stew from #3 and add additional Meat Stock to the pot. Now you have soup! (Soup has more stock in it than a stew.)

Stage 1+ of Intro: Take the soup from #4 and puree it. Now you have a blended or pureed soup!

Stage 1+ of Intro: Strain the Meat Stock and store the liquid in the refrigerator to drink later or use as the basis of a vegetable soup. Pull the meat off the bones, saving bones for Bone Broth as in #2.

Full GAPS diet: You can use the meat for a meat salad with homemade mayonnaise. You can also make gravy with Meat Stock and gelatin, or use it for another entrée.

Meat Stock and Bone Broth

Bone Broth—It's All About the Bones

3

Remember, no Bone Broth until you're on the Full GAPS diet!

To successfully make a gelatinous Bone Broth, you need joints in the pot. Joints equal gelatin! In the case of beef, bison, lamb, or pork, joints are knuckles or necks, but not meaty necks—remember, those are for Meat Stock only. Feet or "trotters" from pigs will also yield a good amount of gelatin, as will a head, if you can get one. For poultry, joints include necks, wings, backs, and feet—but be sure the backs don't have much meat on them. It's also a good idea to cut up the necks, backs, and wings either prior to cooking or after an hour or so in the pot. This will allow the water greater access to the gelatin. The addition of chicken heads will also gel a pot of Bone Broth for you.

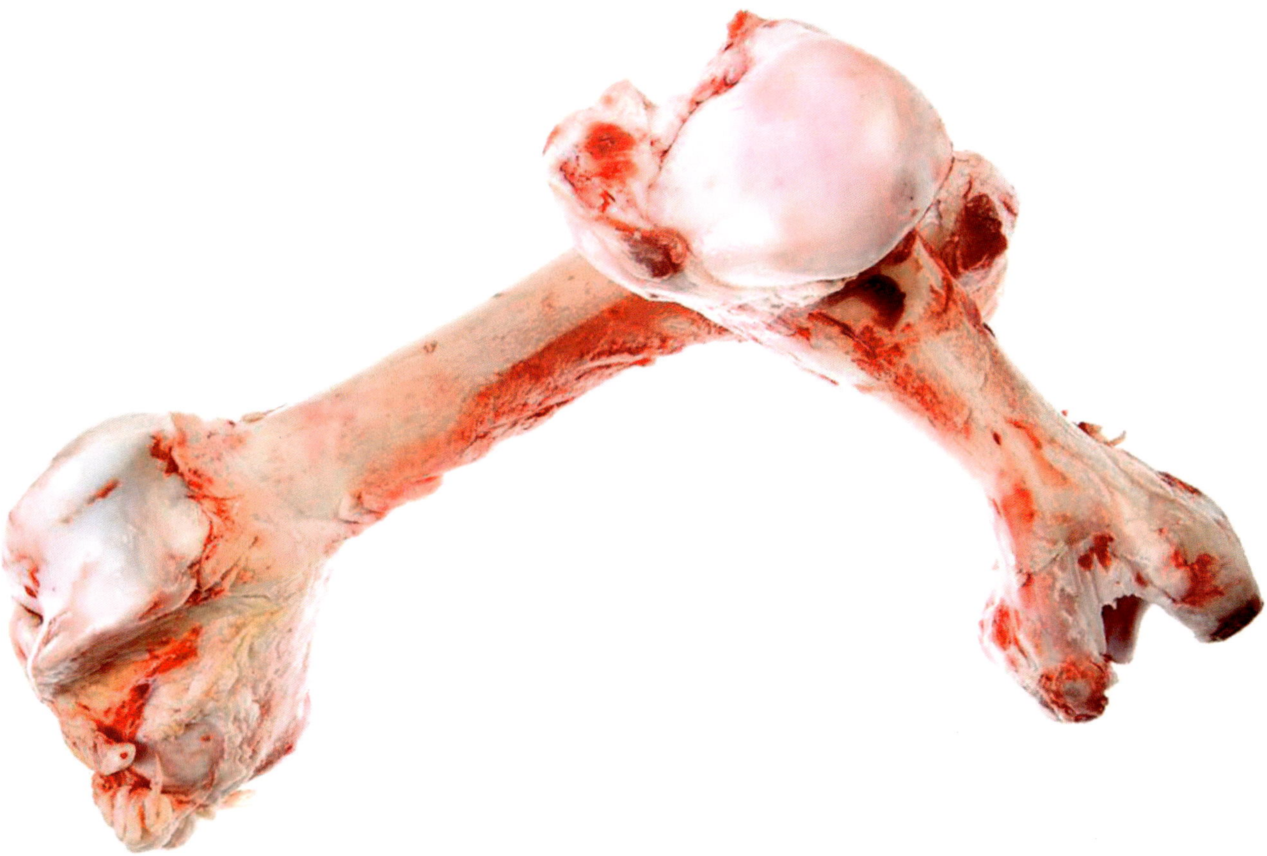

Handy Bone Broth Chart

	Bone Broth: Beef	Bone Broth: Chicken
Bones	Approximately 7 lbs. total: 4 lbs. boney bones for gelatin: marrow and knuckle bones or neck bones that aren't meaty (using more joints than marrow will yield more gelatin) 3 lbs. meaty bones for flavor and color: short ribs, marrow bones with meat on them (also known as "soup bones"), meaty neck bones	1 free range stewing hen or layer, neck and wings cut up (about 3 lbs.) ***or*** 3–4 lbs. boney chicken parts: combination of necks, backs, and wings ***or*** Picked carcasses of 2 chickens (about 4 lbs.) Plus 4 chicken feet and 1 chicken head. Optional, but chicken feet and heads add a lot of gelatin, so use them if you can get them!
Vegetables (organic preferred)	3 celery ribs 3 carrots 3 onions Coarsely chopped	3 celery 2 carrots 1 onion Coarsely chopped
Water	4 quarts or more pure water, to cover	
Vinegar	½ cup apple cider or other mild vinegar	2 tablespoons apple cider or other mild vinegar
Standing time with vinegar	1 hour or longer (no heat)	½ hour or longer (no heat)
Herbs	1 bunch fresh thyme to start 1 bunch fresh parsley with 10 minutes left	1 bunch fresh parsley with 10 minutes left
Pot	Stainless steel 18/8 stockpot, 12 quart or more	Stainless steel 18/8 stockpot, minimum 8 quart
Simmer (or "roll") time	24–72 hours	6–24 hours

A note on simmer time: If you prefer not to keep your stove running continuously, you may wish to use what I call cumulative time. This involves keeping track of the simmer time and then adding it all up. Do this by bringing your Bone Broth to a boil. Skim and discard the scum. Lower to a simmer and start timing. If you need to turn off the heat, just bring the Bone Broth back to a boil when you're ready, then skim and discard the scum. Lower to a simmer and start timing again. Cumulative time is the total amount of time added together. The total time should equal the amount of time in the chart above.

Finishing the Bone Broth

Strain your Bone Broth into a large glass or ceramic bowl or pan. The larger and longer the pan, the more surface area and the faster the cool down. Let Bone Broth come to room temperature on the counter (lightly covered if necessary to protect from dust, bugs, or other airborne contaminants). Once at room temperature, place Bone Broth into the refrigerator to completely cool. It's best to place the bowl or pan on the bottom shelf to ensure against dripping. Discard bones, meat, and vegetables. When Bone Broth gels, remove fat layer to use for cooking. Portion gelled Bone Broth into quart and pint sized containers with a ladle or cup measure. You may freeze it for up to 6 months or refrigerate it for 5–7 days. After 5–7 days in the refrigerator, if you bring it to a boil again you may

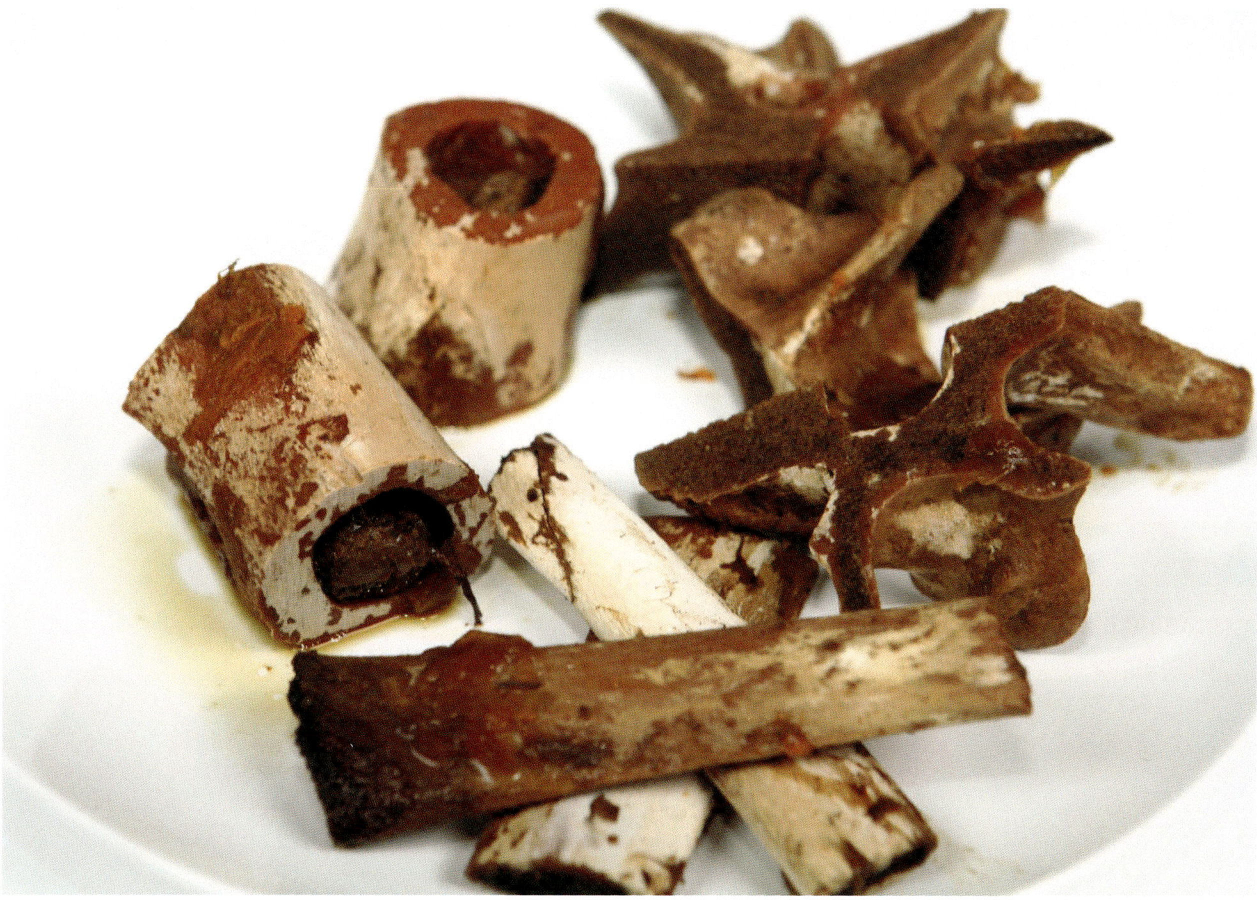

store it for another few days. Exception: If your Bone Broth has been sealed with a layer of tallow, it should keep in the refrigerator for months.

Important Notes Regarding Bone Broth

When using Bone Broth for any recipe, always bring it to a boil, then **skim and discard the scum** before proceeding.

If your Bone Broth fails to gel when cooled, one or more of the following may have occurred:

- Not enough bones with cartilage or connective tissue (joints for beef, or in the case of poultry, feet)
- Too much water to bones
- Too much meat to bones (occurs frequently with chicken)
- Cooked at too high or too low a temperature
- Too much water added while cooking

But don't be discouraged. Even if your Bone Broth didn't gel as it cooled, it's still worth drinking. It's mineral-rich, with electrolytic minerals to boot!

Troubleshooting Bone Broth That Doesn't Gel

A nutrient-dense Bone Broth will gel when cooled. If yours doesn't gel after 24 hours of cooling, you may think about adding a good quality gelatin such as Bernard Jensen's Bovine Gelatin or Great Lakes brand. Store-bought gelatin is made from Bone Broth, so it will also be high in glutamic acid. If you're drinking Bone Broth, it's assumed that your gut is already healed, so this shouldn't be a problem.

Also remember that gelatin is very high in glutamic acid, which can trigger nervous system symptoms if the gut hasn't yet healed. If you add gelatin to your Bone Broth and experience symptoms, you may wish to go back to the Intro diet and Meat Stock. These symptoms are a sign that your gut is still permeable.

Bone Broth Recipes

The following are recipes for Bone Broth. The recipe for beef or bison Bone Broth is the same, as they are both large mammals with large bones. For the chicken Bone Broth, please feel free to use other poultry such as turkey, duck, goose, quail, pheasant, etc. However, due to the fact that turkey bones are larger than chicken or other bones mentioned, you may need to increase the cook time. How to know when a poultry Bone Broth has cooked long enough? All of the connective tissue and cartilage has dissolved into the Broth, and the bones are soft enough that you may crush the ends between your fingers with ease.

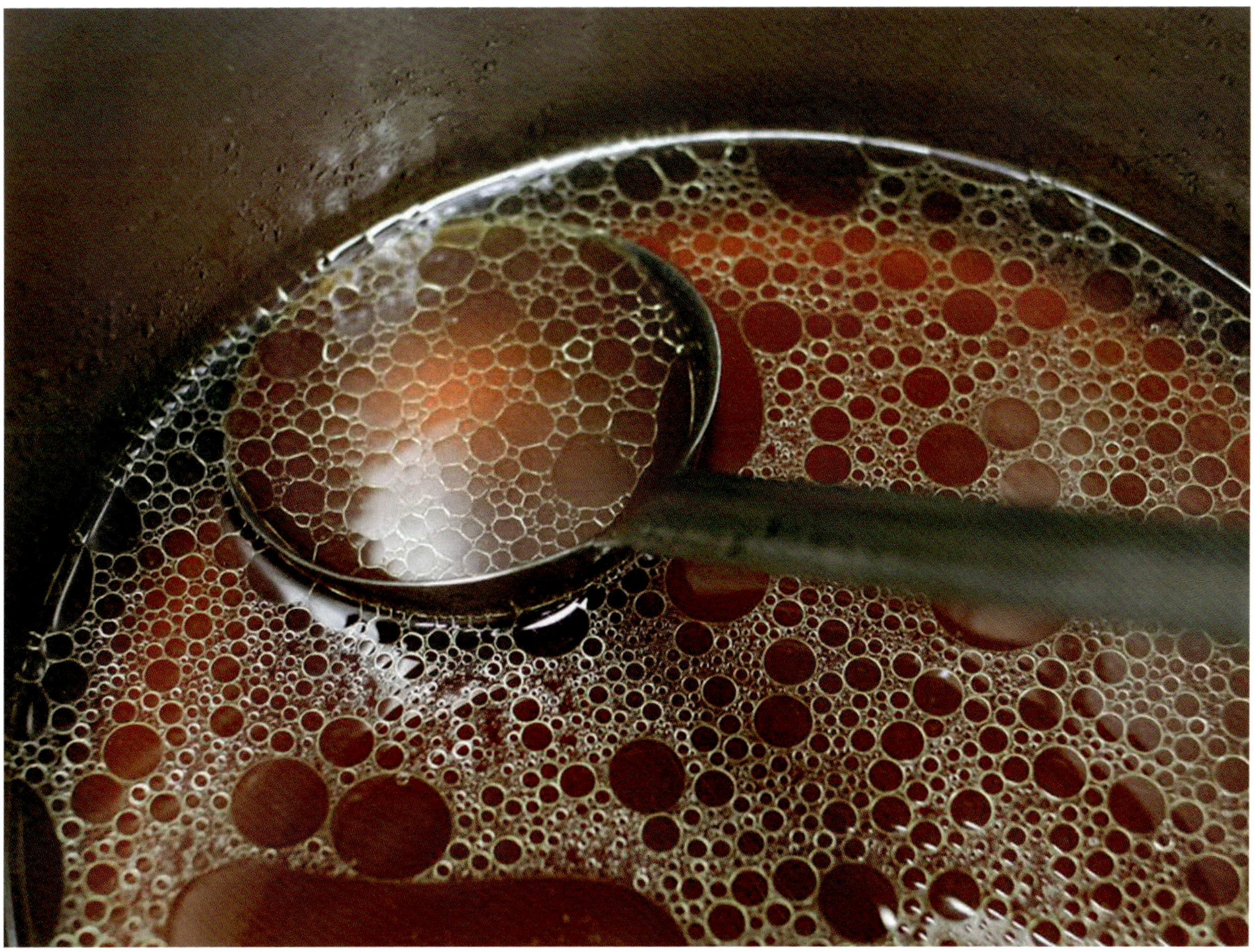

Beef or Bison Bone Broth

Makes about 4 quarts

Ingredients

About 4 lbs. boney bones for gelatin (joints and marrow bones, mostly knuckles and necks)
About 3 lbs. meaty bones (such as ribs) for color and flavor
4 quarts of pure water, or more to cover bones
3 celery ribs, coarsely chopped
3 carrots, coarsely chopped
3 onions, coarsely chopped
½ cup vinegar

Instructions

1. Place meaty bones on a baking sheet lined with parchment paper or a glass pan. Roast in the oven at 350°F until browned, approximately 30 minutes. Meanwhile, place boney bones and all other ingredients in a large, heavy stock pot and leave at room temperature for 1 hour. The vinegar will act on the bones and draw out the calcium and minerals. When the meaty bones are browned, add to the pot along with any accumulated juices.

2. Bring to a boil. Skim and discard the scum, then lower to a rolling simmer for 24–72 hours. This means it should be still on the surface and "rolling" (simmering) underneath.

3. Strain. Bring to room temperature, then cool completely in the refrigerator.

Chicken Bone Broth I: Carcass

Makes about 4 quarts.

Ingredients

- 2 chicken carcasses, picked of meat
- 4 chicken feet and/or 1 chicken head
- 4 quarts pure water
- 3 celery ribs, coarsely chopped
- 2 carrots, coarsely chopped
- 1 onion, coarsely chopped
- 2 tablespoons vinegar

Instructions

1. Place all ingredients in a heavy stockpot and let stand at room temperature for 30 minutes, allowing the vinegar to act on the bones and draw the minerals into the water.
2. Bring the Bone Broth to a boil. Skim and discard the scum. Lower to a simmer. Cover and simmer for 6–24 hours.
3. Strain. Bring to room temperature, then cool completely in the refrigerator.

If your Bone Broth doesn't gel when cooled, see Troubleshooting Bone Broth That Doesn't Gel on page 50.

Chicken Bone Broth II: Layer or Stewing Hen

Makes about 4 quarts

Ingredients

1 layer or stewing hen (about 3 lbs.)
4 chicken feet and/or 1 chicken head
4 quarts pure water
3 celery ribs, coarsely chopped
2 carrots, coarsely chopped
1 onion, coarsely chopped
2 tablespoons vinegar

Instructions

1. Cut the stewing hen up, being sure to cut the neck and wings into several pieces.

2. Place all chicken pieces except feet and head on a parchment-lined sheet pan. Roast the pieces in the oven at 350°F for about 20-30 minutes, until golden brown.

3. For next steps, follow instructions for Chicken Bone Broth I.

Chicken Bone Broth III: Necks, Backs, and Wings

Makes about 4 quarts

Ingredients

4 lbs. necks, backs (not meaty), and/or wings, cut up
4 chicken feet and/or 1 chicken head
4 quarts pure water
3 celery ribs, coarsely chopped
2 carrots, coarsely chopped
1 onion, coarsely chopped
2 tablespoons vinegar

Instructions

1. Place all chicken pieces except feet and head on a parchment-lined sheet pan.

2. Roast chicken pieces at 350°F for about 20-30 minutes, until golden brown.

3. For next steps, follow instructions for Chicken Bone Broth I.

Important Facts About Bone Broth

What's the role of vinegar in Bone Broth? You may have noticed there's no vinegar in Meat Stock, but there is in Bone Broth. Why? The role of vinegar is to draw or leach the minerals out of the bones and into the Bone Broth. Meat Stock is full of meat, and the bones are covered with meat, so the vinegar cannot act on them.

Temperature counts. How do you know your Bone Broth is cooking at the right temperature? The best way is to check the movement as it simmers. It should be relatively still on the top, but you should see movement underneath. If the temperature is too high or too low, the Bone Broth won't gel.

Don't bother eating the meat or vegetables from the Bone Broth. Not only will they be tasteless and mushy, but they're spent of nutrients as well. They've given everything into the Bone Broth, and now they're just a shadow of what they used to be. But their flavors, minerals, and nutrients remain in the Bone Broth.

To cool or not to cool your Bone Broth? I'm often asked if it's safe to leave a pot of Bone Broth on the stove in between cook times, as I suggest when using cumulative time. Should you put the pot in the refrigerator when you leave the house or leave it on the stove? If you put a hot pot into a cold refrigerator, your Bone Broth actually has a **greater** chance of growing putrefying or opportunistic bacteria. You also run the risk of spoiling the food in your fridge and making it work very hard to bring the temperature back to where it should be. Here are good rules of thumb to guide you:

You can safely leave a pot of Bone Broth on the stove as long as you bring it to a boil and skim the scum once every 12 hours.

If you're going to be away from your Bone Broth for 24 or more hours, cool it to room temperature first, and then place it in the refrigerator. When you return, bring the pot to a boil, skim and discard any scum, turn the pot down to a simmer. Cover and continue cooking.

Bone Broth is sustainable. Bone Broth is very much part of a sustainable living paradigm. Save the bones from your Meat Stock in the freezer until you're ready to make Bone Broth. That is, **after** your gut is healed from the Intro diet.

Cost-cutting hint: save your veggies! Whenever you cook, always freeze the ends of celery, carrots, and onions (including skins), in a freezer-proof bag or container. When you go to make Bone Broth, you won't have to go out and purchase the vegetables because you'll already have what you need.

Meat Stock and Bone Broth

Everything Else You Need to Know

4

From cooking with slow cookers to storing your Bone Broth, here are a few more helpful hints.

About Slow Cookers

What about using a slow cooker for making Meat Stock or Bone Broth? They're ideal for Meat Stock, but not so good for Bone Broth. Why? Slow cookers don't get hot enough to bring Bone Broth to a boil. (Remember that whole Bring it to a boil and skim and discard the scum thing?) Slow cookers also

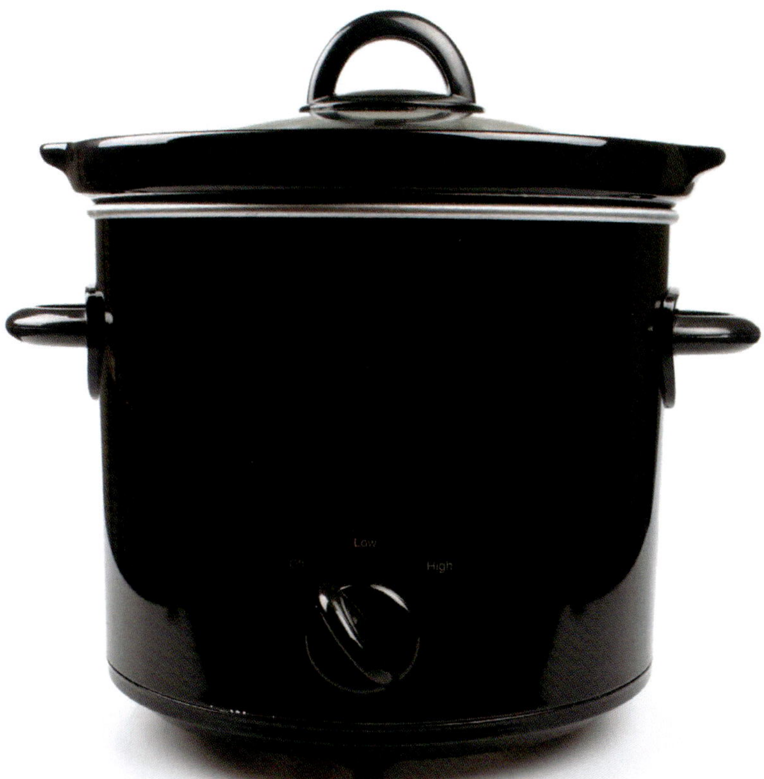

aren't big enough, generally, to hold Beef Bone Broth: 7 lbs. of bones and vegetables, plus 4 quarts of water.

On the other hand, slow cookers are great for Meat Stock: 2–3 lbs. of meaty bones, vegetables, and water to cover. You'll still need to extend your cooking time if you use a slow cooker for Meat Stock because it takes a while for the slow cooker to come up to temperature. See the Handy Meat Stock Chart on page 42 for time considerations.

There's one other thing to consider about slow cookers: the research that determined how much glutamic acid was in Meat Stock and Bone Broth wasn't done using a slow cooker. If you're highly sensitive to glutamic acid, it may be best for you to use a Dutch oven and skip the slow cooker. See "Comparative Analysis of Amino Acids in Short Cooked Chicken Meat Stock and Long Cooked Chicken Bone Broth" on page 40.

The Quality of the Meat, Bones, and Water

The Gut and Psychology Syndrome is a healing protocol. Therefore, use the best quality food you can find. If the gut is already leaking, the body will have its share of toxins to deal with because of it. Using clean meat, bones, and vegetables will not add to that already toxic load. Your ingredients count, so make it real food: organic food, food you grow yourself, or food from a farmer you trust. Use meat and bones from animals raised on pasture their entire lives. That means grass-fed *and* grass-finished. This will keep GMO soy and corn out of your diet—because it wasn't in theirs. And by the way, no soy is allowed on the GAPS diet—that goes for both the Intro and Full GAPS diet. **Nada.**

As for the water you use to make Meat Stock or Bone Broth, it's very important that it be pure. Spring water is best. If you use distilled water or reverse osmosis (RO), water, be sure to add minerals to it before you begin. A good source is ConcenTrace Trace Minerals.

Pots: Which for Which?

Meat Stock is prepared in a Dutch oven, a large, heavy pot made of cast iron or cast iron and porcelain, with a tight lid. Dutch ovens are used for slow cooking, usually stews and braising. They can be used on the stovetop or in the oven. If you don't have a Dutch oven, you may use a 6–8 quart stockpot. However, you can only use it on the stove.

Bone Broth is prepared in a stockpot. The best stockpots are made of 18/8 stainless steel. They're tall and thin, with a narrow opening. The small opening means less surface area, which translates into less evaporation—you will lose less of your Bone Broth due to evaporation. I also highly recommend a glass lid because it lets you see if your Bone Broth is simmering at the correct temperature.

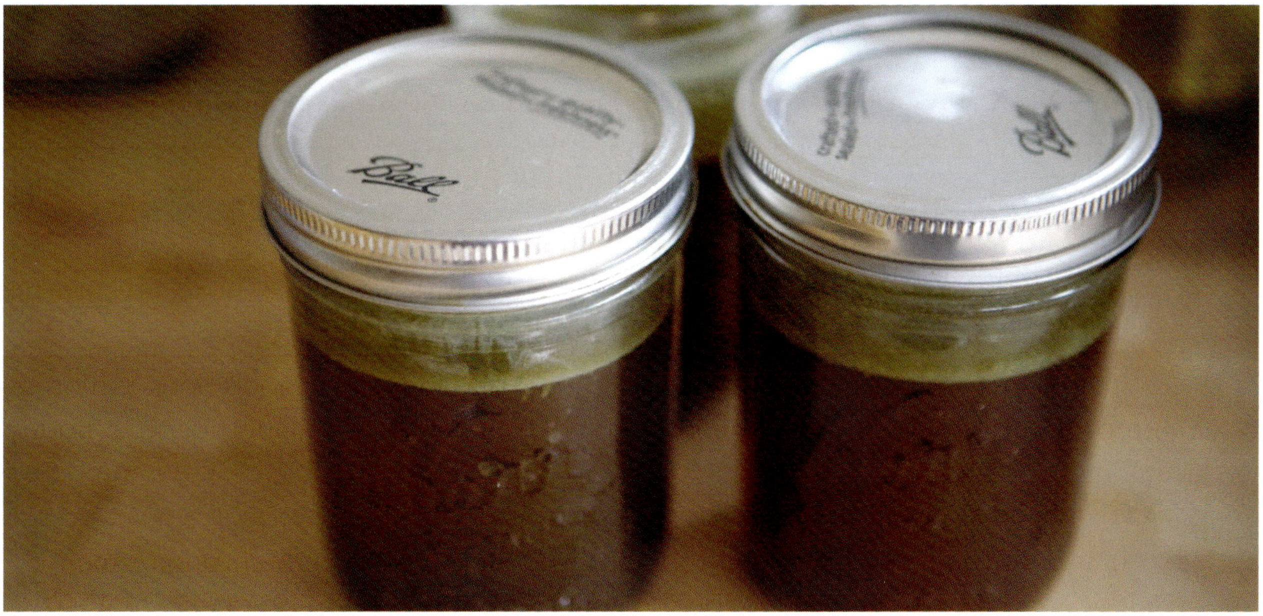

Storing Options for Bone Broth

You may also use some of the following options for storing Meat Stock, but in general you'll be eating and drinking your Meat Stock as you make it, and therefore you won't need to store it.

Here are three great storage options for Bone Broth:

Store in a glass jar in the refrigerator. If a layer of fat forms on top, it will seal out any air and keep for several months. If there is no layer of fat, the Bone Broth will last 5–7 days in the refrigerator. After this time, bring it to a boil, then skim and discard any scum. Once it cools, it will keep in the refrigerator for a few more days.

Store in a glass jar in the freezer. Freezer-safe canning jars have straight sides that prevent them from cracking in the freezer. If you choose this option, leave 2 inches of space at the top of the jar, don't tighten the lid until the liquid has frozen, and make sure the jars don't touch in the freezer. To defrost, place the glass jar in the refrigerator for a few days. To speed up the thawing process, you may gently submerge the frozen glass jar in a bowl or sink filled with cold water. Just be careful you don't rush it, or you'll have a broken jar on your hands!

Make Bone Broth ice cubes. Once your Bone Broth is at room temperature, pour into ice cube trays and freeze it. Remove frozen cubes from the tray and store them in a container or bag in the freezer for ease of use. This is a nice way to make a cup or two of Bone Broth for drinking—simply heat up a cube or two for a mug.

If you must use plastic for storage, be sure it's BPA free. Also, you may wish to line the plastic container with parchment paper so the Bone Broth doesn't come into contact with the plastic. Never pour hot Bone Broth or any other hot liquid into a plastic container. Plastic contains chemicals that leach into food. Wait until it has cooled to at least room temperature.

Don't store hot broth or stock in plastic! Plastic contains chemicals that leach into food.

Which Fats Are Healthy and Why?

Dr. Natasha Campbell-McBride is very clear that saturated animal fats are optimal for human health and healing. As such, they're a large part of the GAPS diet, and you should use them liberally while implementing the diet. Traditional animal fats are safe for cooking because they don't change their structure when heated. These fats include tallow from beef, lamb, or bison, lard from pigs, schmaltz from chickens, duck or goose fat, etc. Though not optimal, you may also use coconut oil because it's a healthy saturated fat from the vegetable kingdom. Virgin, cold-pressed olive oil is a monounsaturated fat and also healthful, but it should only be consumed cold or at room temperature, never heated. Note that olive oil is not included until Stage 4 of the Intro.

Which Salt Is Good Salt? Why Does It Matter?

It's very important to use good quality salt for Meat Stock and for the GAPS diet in general, as most people on the GAPS diet have mineral deficiencies. Good quality means no fillers or anti-caking agents, and the packaging should list the amount of trace minerals in the salt. I look for a minimum of 50 trace minerals or more. Sea salt is usually the best because it provides a broad spectrum of minerals in good quantity.

No Microwaves Allowed!

Microwaves are not allowed on the GAPS diet. Do not use microwaves to reheat Meat Stock or Bone Broth. Dr. Natasha Campbell-McBride has been very clear that "microwaves destroy food."

Section VIII | Culturing Dairy

Foreword

> Another good book by Monica Corrado! She gives a good overall explanation about dairy products and how to use them correctly to regain your health. I warmly recommend it!
>
> Humans consumed fermented milk products for thousands of years. They are an excellent way to nourish your body and restore not only your gut flora but also the microbial flora on your skin, scalp, and mucous membranes. By applying homemade kefir and sour cream on any problem area on your body, you can soothe and heal that area. These foods provide nourishing substances for your skin and mucous membranes as well as probiotic microbes.
>
> Of course, we are talking about homemade, high-quality fermented dairy. That means fresh, organic, unprocessed milk from animals who live the way Mother Nature designed them to live—on pasture, on fresh grass, and under the sunlight. Monica's guidance makes it easy to learn how to make these healing foods for yourself and your family. Once you start using fermented dairy products, you and your family won't want to be without them anymore!
>
> —Dr. Natasha Campbell-McBride

Culturing Dairy
Introduction

Cultured dairy is a large part of the Gut and Psychology Syndrome (GAPS) diet. Some people shy away from the diet because they have dairy allergies or sensitivities, yet the GAPS healing protocol is designed precisely to help clear up the cause of such sensitivities.

Allergies and sensitivities are symptoms of a "leaky gut," a damaged small intestine that is unable to either break down food or absorb nutrients the food would provide. The Gut and Psychology Syndrome diet is designed to heal and seal the damaged area of the small intestine (the duodenum). This takes place during the Intro diet, especially with the consumption of Meat Stock, as explained in the previous section. So to be clear, the "healing and sealing" of the gut lining takes place in the Intro diet of the GAPS diet by eating Meat Stock.

As you may know, most people have dairy "sensitivities" rather than true allergies. Symptoms of a dairy sensitivity can include bloating, constipation, gas, or cramping. Other symptoms may be eczema or a skin rash, bright red ears after eating a suspect food, a runny nose, or chronic sinus infections. You may have a sensitivity either to the lactose (milk sugar) or to the casein (a type of protein) found in dairy. If you have been tested for a true dairy allergy, which is a reaction to the protein in milk, you may be wary of this part of the protocol. No need to fear: whether you are sensitive or allergic, there is help for you here! The Dairy Introduction Protocol was developed for just this reason. It is a simple, specifically timed, step-by-step introduction of certain types of cultured dairy into your diet, starting with dairy that is the easiest to digest.

> **Symptoms of lactose intolerance:** Some people are "lactose intolerant." Symptoms of lactose intolerance include diarrhea, bloating, flatulence or gas, constipation, cramping, or general malaise. When dairy is cultured for a minimum of 24 hours, nearly all of the lactose will be predigested (or eliminated), and the symptoms will be gone too!

Culturing Dairy

What Is "Dairy" and Why Culture It?

1

For our purposes dairy is milk or cream that comes from cows, goats, or sheep. Some people are even drinking camel milk these days in an effort to find proteins they can tolerate. Different species have different protein structures, so you may find it difficult to tolerate the proteins found in cow milk but not in goat or sheep milk. Yet even different breeds of cows have different protein structures. For example, in recent years we have learned

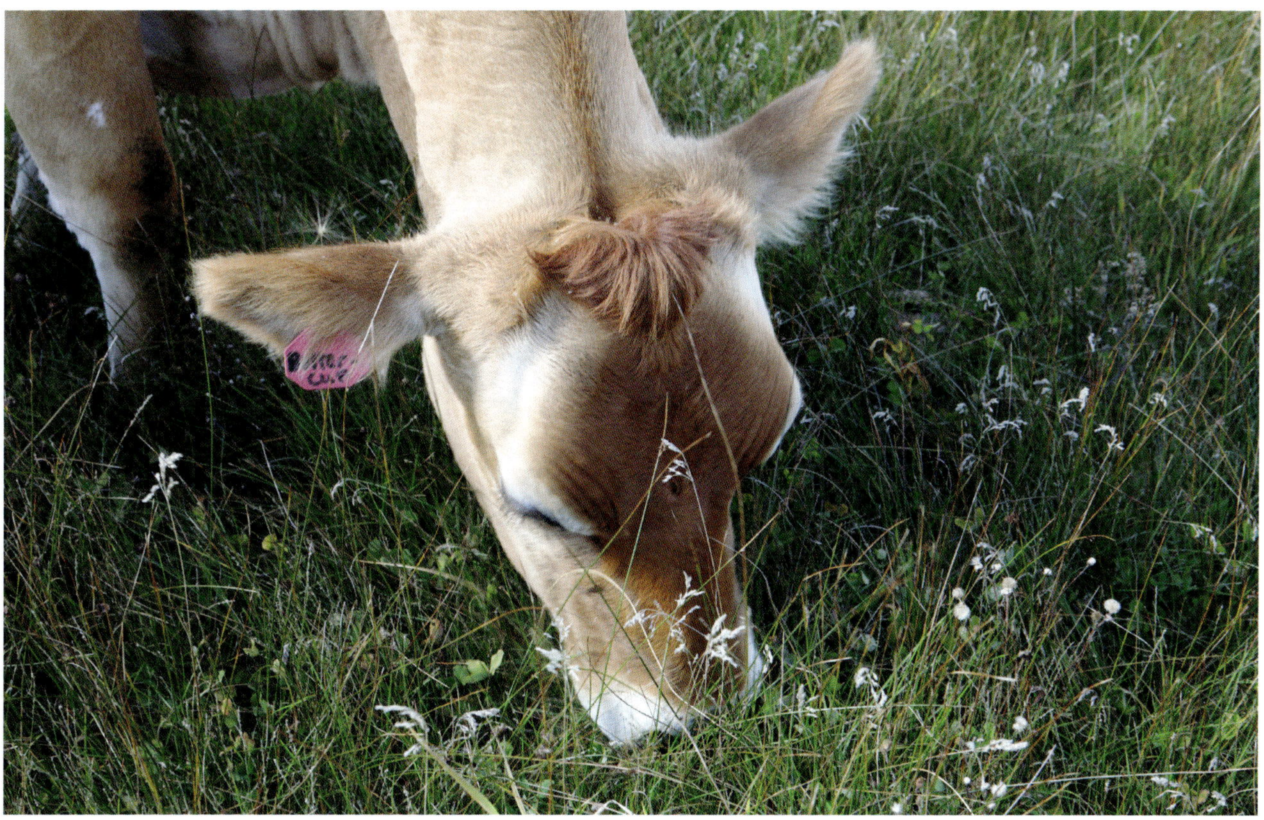

that the A1 milk protein from black-and-white Holsteins is problematic for many people but most notably for those on the autism spectrum. Yet the A2 protein found in milk from brown cows such as Guernseys or Jerseys is much more digestible for the majority of people.

For more information on A1 and A2 milk:

> See the slideshow "Beta-Casomorphin-7 and A1, A2 Milk: The Devil's in the Details" (http://windsordairy.com/casomorphine.html) by Meg Cattell, DVM, MS.
>
> Read the book *Devil in the Milk: Illness, Health and the Politics of A1 and A2 Milk* by Keith Woodford.

Dr. Natasha Campbell-McBride strongly suggests that we use only milk from brown cows for the GAPS diet, and that those cows be grass-fed. This milk is rich in vitamin D and does not contain the problematic proteins.

Liquid milk can be hard to digest even in its most natural state: fresh from the cow, otherwise known as "raw." But pasteurized milk is *always* hard on the digestive tract. When you culture milk or cream for a minimum of 24 hours, you make it easier to digest. Culturing predigests the lactose and partially digests the casein, a long-chain protein found in milk. These proteins and sugars are predigested for you by "good" bacteria, or cultures. You know them as probiotics; I call them "gut good guys." Culturing dairy adds probiotics and increases live enzymes, factors that result in more efficient digestion.

To be clear, when you implement the Gut and Psychology Syndrome healing protocol or diet, you must culture dairy for the following reasons:

- To break down or predigest the lactose, a milk sugar that would otherwise feed opportunistic or putrefying bacteria and contribute to continued gut dysbiosis and toxins in the bloodstream.
- To partially break down casein, a long-chain protein found in milk that the body cannot use until it is broken down or digested. A damaged small intestine does not have the capacity to digest casein, which would continue to damage the small intestine lining due to its size.
- To break down casein so it does not enter the bloodstream as casomorphin, which acts as an opiate and is toxic to brain function. (Casomorphin is one of the first stages of digested casein. If you culture dairy as outlined in this section, casein will break down past this stage.)
- To add live enzymes, which stimulate the digestion process and help digest the food you eat.
- To gain beneficial bacterial cultures and yeast (see list below).
- To add lactic acid (contributed by lactobacilli) to the digestive tract.

You *must* culture dairy for a minimum of 24 hours to ensure that lactose, a sugar found in milk, breaks down prior to consumption. I often leave my milk or cream to culture on the counter for 36 hours, just to be sure.

Please note that all of the techniques in this section may be used to culture milk from cows, goats, sheep—and even camels, if desired. If you have a known intolerance to dairy products, Dr. Natasha often suggests starting with goat milk when you begin culturing dairy.

We love "good" bacteria to culture dairy (and yeast and bacteria to culture kefir) because they:

- Render dairy easier to digest.
- Maintain the health of the small intestine.
- Make us more resistant to illness.
- Aid overall digestion.
- Make the nutrients in dairy more available to the body.
- Increase the vitamin B and C content of milk.
- Create vitamins such as B12 and a form of vitamin K.
- Contribute lactic acid, which is healing and soothing to the gut. Lactic acid feeds the intestinal flora that keeps *Candida albicans* in check.

Culturing Dairy

Which Milk Is Best? Why?

2

Fresh, raw milk from Guernsey and Jersey cows is best. RealMilk.com can help you find more information on locating raw milk near you. If you cannot obtain certified raw milk, the next best is organic, whole, grass-fed, nonhomogenized milk.

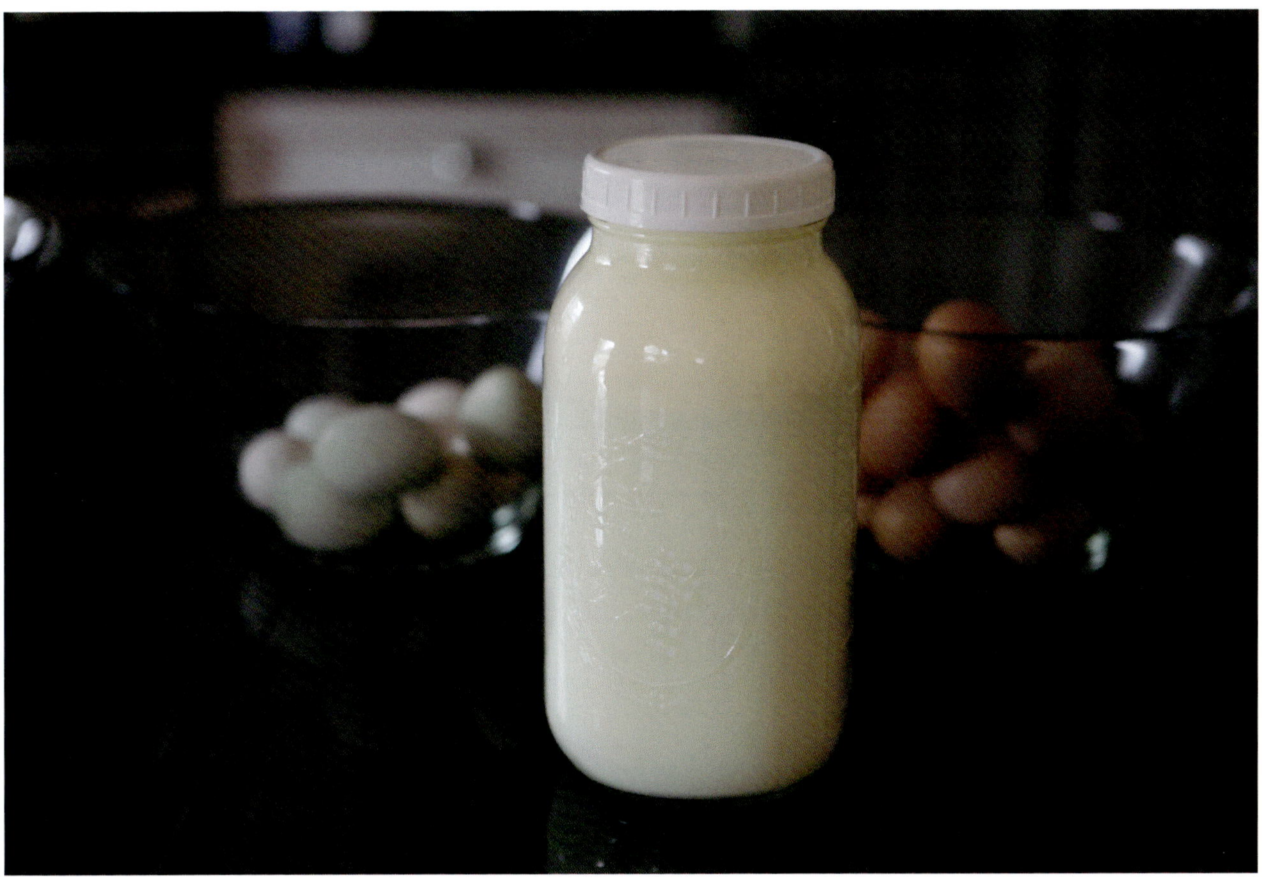

Here are some more detailed guidelines to follow if you must use pasteurized milk:

- Always use organic milk. These cows have not eaten conventional feed that is almost sure to contain GMO soy and corn. Soy and corn are not allowed on the diet, and GMOs are certainly prohibited. Buying organic also ensures that the cows have not been administered antibiotics or growth hormones. Organic does not guarantee that the milk is from grass-fed, pasture-raised cows, which provides superior nutrient quality. Think of organic as a safeguard against things you do not want in your dairy. Unfortunately it does not mean nutrient rich.
- Purchase organic milk from grass-fed cows as they produce superior, nutrient rich milk. This is the milk that nature intended, and you do not have to worry the cow ate corn or soy, which are not permitted in the diet.
- Look for milk that has been pasteurized at low temperatures. The label will state "low temperature pasteurized."
- Do not use ultra-pasteurized or ultra-high-temperature (UHT) pasteurized milk. It has been denatured too strongly, and it will not support a culture. And who knows what grows in it—so just do not use it.
- Always use whole or full-fat milk as you cannot absorb calcium or vitamins A and D without fat. (GAPS patients and those who are healing their guts *need* extra fat, so no skimping with skim.)

An important note about raw milk: Keep in mind that as you go through the GAPS diet, you need to gradually add cultured dairy products *before* you consume raw milk. Dr. Natasha suggests that you wait one year after completing the Intro diet before adding raw milk and/or raw cream to your diet.

Handy Milk Buying Guide

Best	Acceptable (Not Optimal)	Acceptable (Less Optimal)	Not Recommended	Worst
Fresh, raw milk from pasture-raised cows	Organic, pasteurized, nonhomogenized milk from grass-fed cows	Organic, pasteurized, homogenized milk	Organic, UHT pasteurized milk that does not support live cultures	Conventional milk

Culturing Dairy

Why Homemade Cultured Dairy Products?

3

If at all possible, it is important to make your own cultured dairy products for the Gut and Psychology Syndrome healing protocol. There are three important reasons for doing so.

1. When you make your own cultured dairy products, you ensure the quality of the ingredients you ingest. This is a healing protocol, so it is important to use the highest quality ingredients you can find. As previously stated, the American dairy industry uses inferior A1 milk from black-

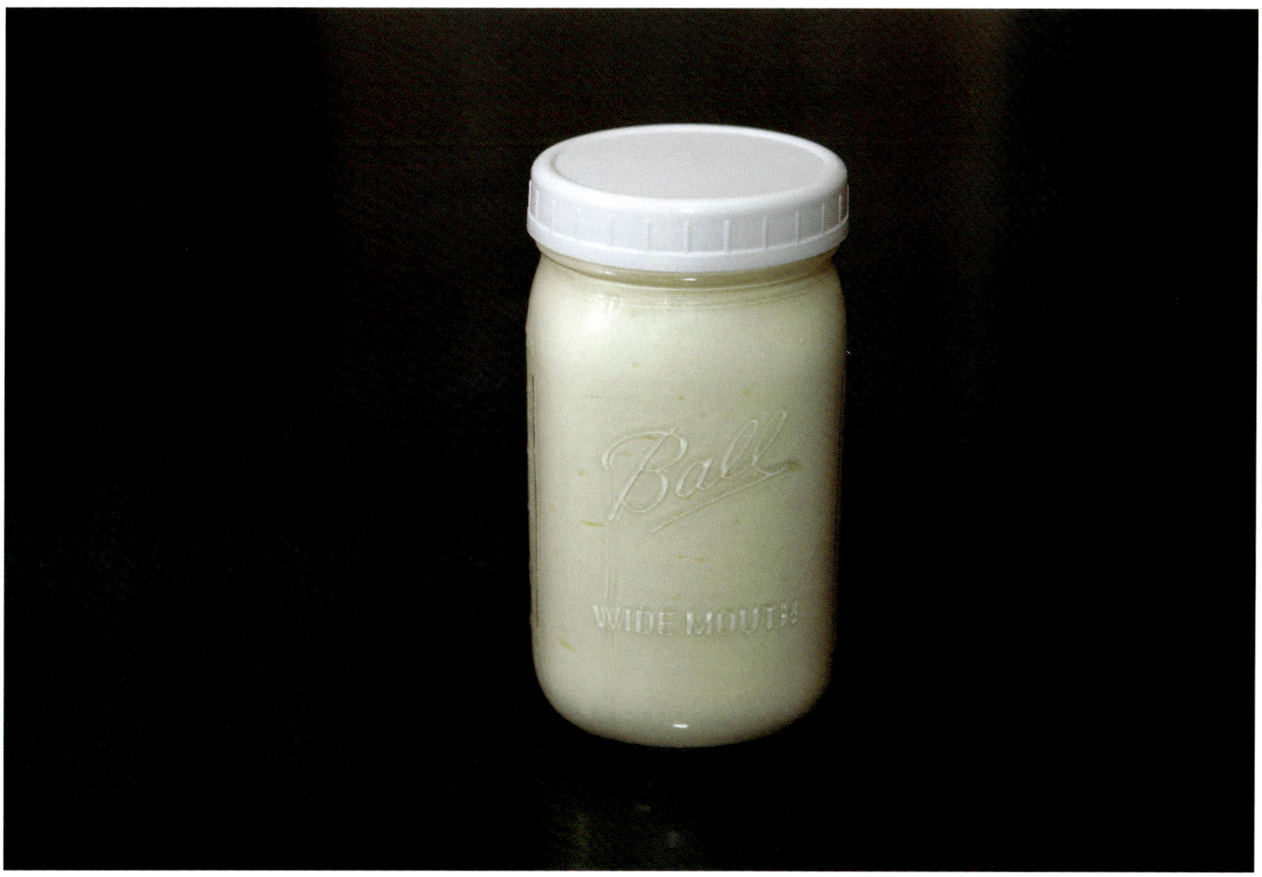

and-white Holsteins, and the vast majority of cultured dairy products available commercially—organic or not—are produced from this milk.

2. Most commercially available yogurt and kefir contains pectin or other additives, including guar gum and/or carrageenan. These ingredients are not permitted on the GAPS diet, but they also point to the inferiority of the milk and whether or not it is organic. Inferior quality milk low in butterfat will not firm up as milk with more butterfat does, which is why pectin, guar gum, and carrageenan are added in the first place.

3. Commercially available crème fraîche, yogurt, and kefir are cultured for a short amount of time, sometimes for as little as 6 hours. This is not enough time for the culturing process to predigest the problematic lactose, so the dairy will still contain it. Lactose is not permitted on the GAPS diet for the reasons noted above.

A note about sour cream: Dr. Natasha includes sour cream in her book *Gut and Psychology Syndrome*. However, real, pure sour(ed) cream is not commercially available in the United States (see below). We use crème fraîche instead. If you have access to raw cream, see the recipe for making sour cream in chapter 7 and include it in your diet. Remember to keep in mind that sour cream can *only* be made from *raw* cream.

American Sour Cream Is Not Really Sour Cream

There is no true commercially available sour cream in the United States at this time. Real sour cream is cream that has been left to sour, and one would *never* allow pasteurized cream to sour—it would make you very sick! Remember, pasteurization is sterilization, and a sterile environment is a breeding ground for putrefying or opportunistic bacteria to grow. All of the "sour cream" you currently find in stores is pasteurized cream that has been cultured—so it is actually "cultured cream." Or, as the French call it, "crème fraîche." Sadly, this "sour cream" also contains fillers that are not allowed on the GAPS diet.

Culturing Dairy

To Introduce or Not to Introduce Dairy—Knowing When and How

4

In the Intro diet, dairy is introduced right from the start, in Stage 1, as long as there is no known or suspected sensitivity or allergy. You begin with ghee, butter, whey, crème fraîche, sour cream (if you make it yourself from raw cream), yogurt, and kefir.

If you have a known dairy allergy or concern, do a Skin Sensitivity Test prior to introducing dairy to your diet. It is important to do a test before you introduce each new dairy product.

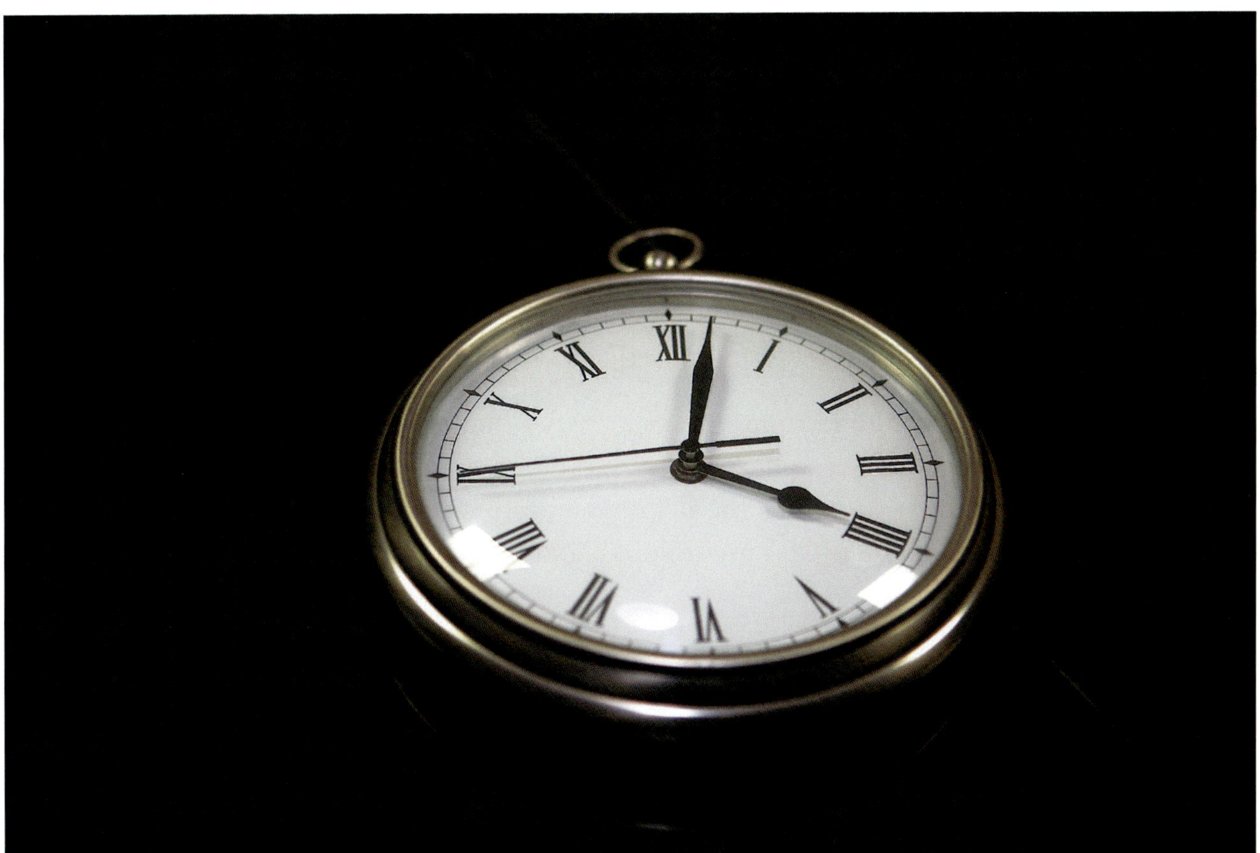

The Skin Sensitivity Test: What It Is, When to Use It, and How to Do It

As I discussed in Section III, the Skin Sensitivity Test (or Sensitivity Test from here forward) tells you if you have a sensitivity to a certain food. It is very easy to do yourself at home—and far less expensive than a battery of allergy tests would be.

Again, use a Sensitivity Test if you have a known allergy or suspect a sensitivity to a food. Most individuals have reactions to protein, so they will not react to ghee or butter (ghee is pure fat, and butter may only have traces of whey in it).

How to do a Sensitivity Test: Place a drop of the food in question (mash solid food with a bit of water) on the inside of the wrist at bedtime. Let the drop dry on the skin (you may wish to cover it with a Band-Aid to keep it there). In the morning, check the spot. If there is a red reaction—what Dr. Natasha calls "an angry red spot"—avoid the food for a few weeks and then try again. If there is no reaction, you may introduce the food gradually, starting with a very small amount.

What is a small amount? A small amount is a *small* amount! When you introduce a food that you have taken out of the diet, or a food you may have been sensitive to, start with a *very small* amount. That means an amount that would fit on the head of a pin. Do not rush to introduce new foods. Slow and steady, inch by inch (or pinhead by pinhead, as the case may be) is always best. Watch to see if the new food triggers any symptoms. If it does, either discontinue the food or hold at the level where the symptom occurred until it passes. At that point, you may slowly increase the amount of the food that triggered the symptom. Proceed with care and attentiveness!

Culturing Dairy

The Dairy Introduction Protocol for Those Who Are Sensitive

5

If you detected a sensitivity to dairy products after doing the Skin Sensitivity Test, the Dairy Introduction Protocol will help you reintroduce these products. *According to Dr. Natasha, those who went straight to the Full GAPS diet and skipped the Intro diet did not heal and seal their gut, so they are also encouraged to do the Dairy Introduction Protocol while on Full GAPS.* They should go dairy-free for about six weeks and then start the Protocol. Purchase only *organic* milk if you're using commercially produced milk. But best is always fresh, raw milk from grass-fed brown cows (Guernseys and Jerseys).

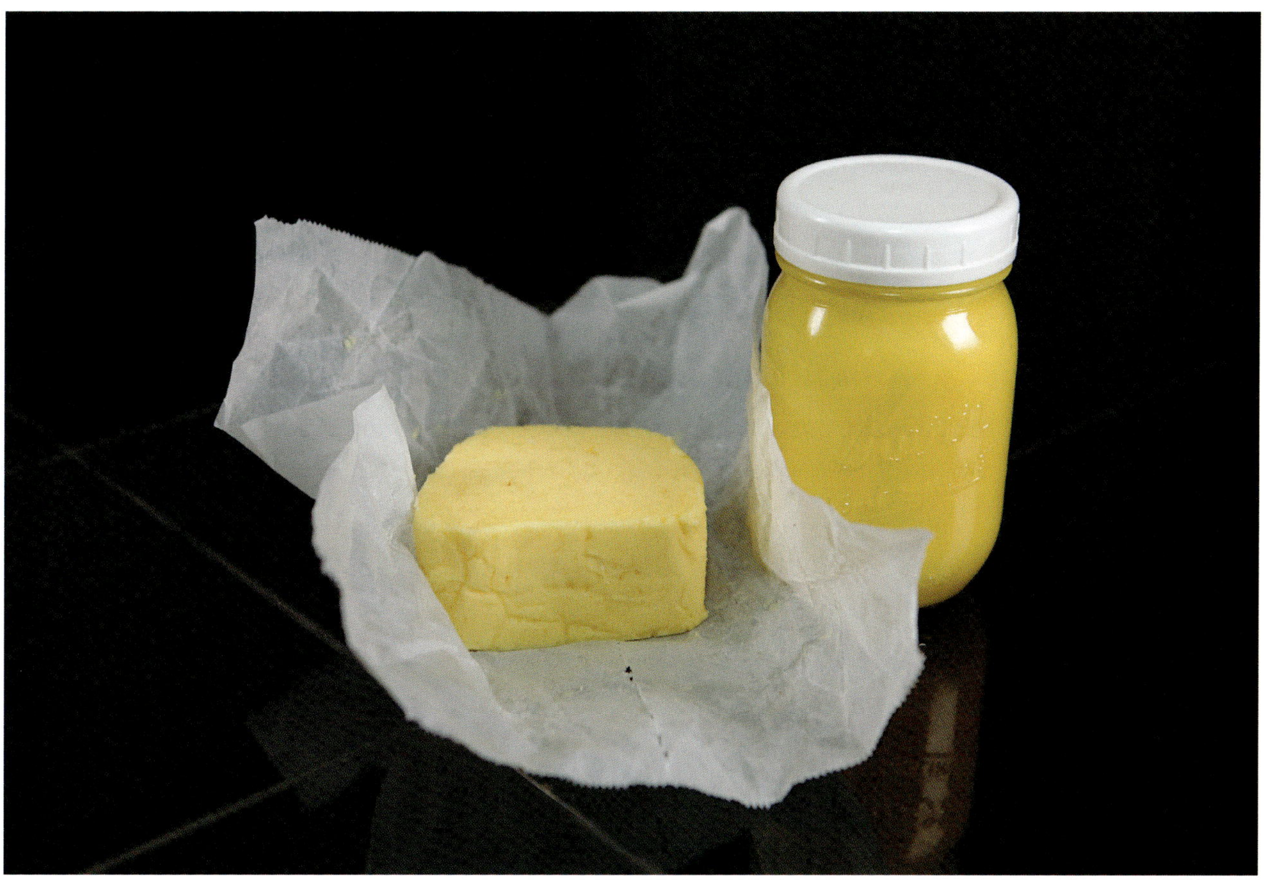

Your Timing Is Your Timing! Do Not Rush Through the Protocol!

Everyone's body is different; therefore, the time it takes to heal or add in a new food is unique to you. Take the time you need. You may be healing decades of damage. It took a while to get to this state—it may take a bit of time to clear it up.

Introduce these foods in the following order, for the amount of time indicated. The order is based on the ease with which these foods are normally introduced to most bodies. The challenge to the digestive system (based on the relative complexity of the molecules) increases by stage, beginning with the most easily digested dairy products and gradually introducing those that are more complex. Dairy fat such as ghee and butter are usually tolerated with ease by most individuals, even those who are very sensitive.

Please note that "tolerating" a new food means you remain symptom-free when eating it. If you experience your typical symptoms (bloating, cramping, gas, constipation, or brain fog for that matter), wait until the symptoms clear before adding the next food. Listen to your body. It will tell you when to add the next food into your diet. Once you add a new food, keep it in your diet. The idea is to keep increasing the types and amounts of foods you can eat.

Dairy Introduction Protocol: Step by Step

1. **Ghee**. This is pure milk fat that contains no lactose or casein. If ghee is tolerated, 6 weeks later, introduce:

2. **Butter from grass-fed cows**. Butter is pure milk fat and a little whey (a simple milk protein, much easier to digest than casein). If butter is tolerated, 6–12 weeks later introduce other cultured dairy products in the order below. Take your time doing this. Note: Each step may take 6–12 weeks, depending on the relative health of your digestive tract and the pace your body is comfortable with. Remember, symptoms such as bloating, constipation, or diarrhea are your body's way of saying, "Let's slow down."

3. **Homemade crème fraîche**. High in fat, homemade crème fraîche is easy to tolerate. It contains milk protein but no lactose if cultured for 24 hours or more. Start with 1 teaspoon per day and increase to 1–2 cups per day.

4. **Homemade yogurt**. Yogurt is a high protein dairy that is a bit more challenging to tolerate. Homemade yogurt will not contain lactose if cultured for a minimum of 24 hours. Start with 1 teaspoon per day and increase to 1–2 cups per day.

5. **Homemade kefir.** Start by making homemade kefir with cream only. After you can tolerate it, prepare kefir with a mixture of cream and milk. And finally, when you

are ready, make kefir with milk only. Homemade kefir made from milk is high in protein, and it may cause constipation in those who are prone to it. Kefir introduces lactic acid-producing yeast in addition to lactic acid-producing bacteria. Yeast can provoke a detox reaction if introduced too early or in too great amount, so take care when you introduce your homemade kefir.

6. **Cheese**. Start with hard cheeses such as cheddar and Parmesan that have been aged for a long time—a minimum of 6 months is best. Eat one mouthful of cheese with a meal. Wait 3–5 days to see if you have a reaction. If no reaction, continue with cheese and all the other dairy foods you have successfully added to your diet.

Culturing Dairy

Dairy, Constipation, and Diarrhea, Oh My!

6

Different bodies respond differently to dairy products. In general that means some people will tend to have loose bowel movements, and some people will tend to have firm bowel movements. If you pay attention to your body and look back over time, you will know which description best fits you.

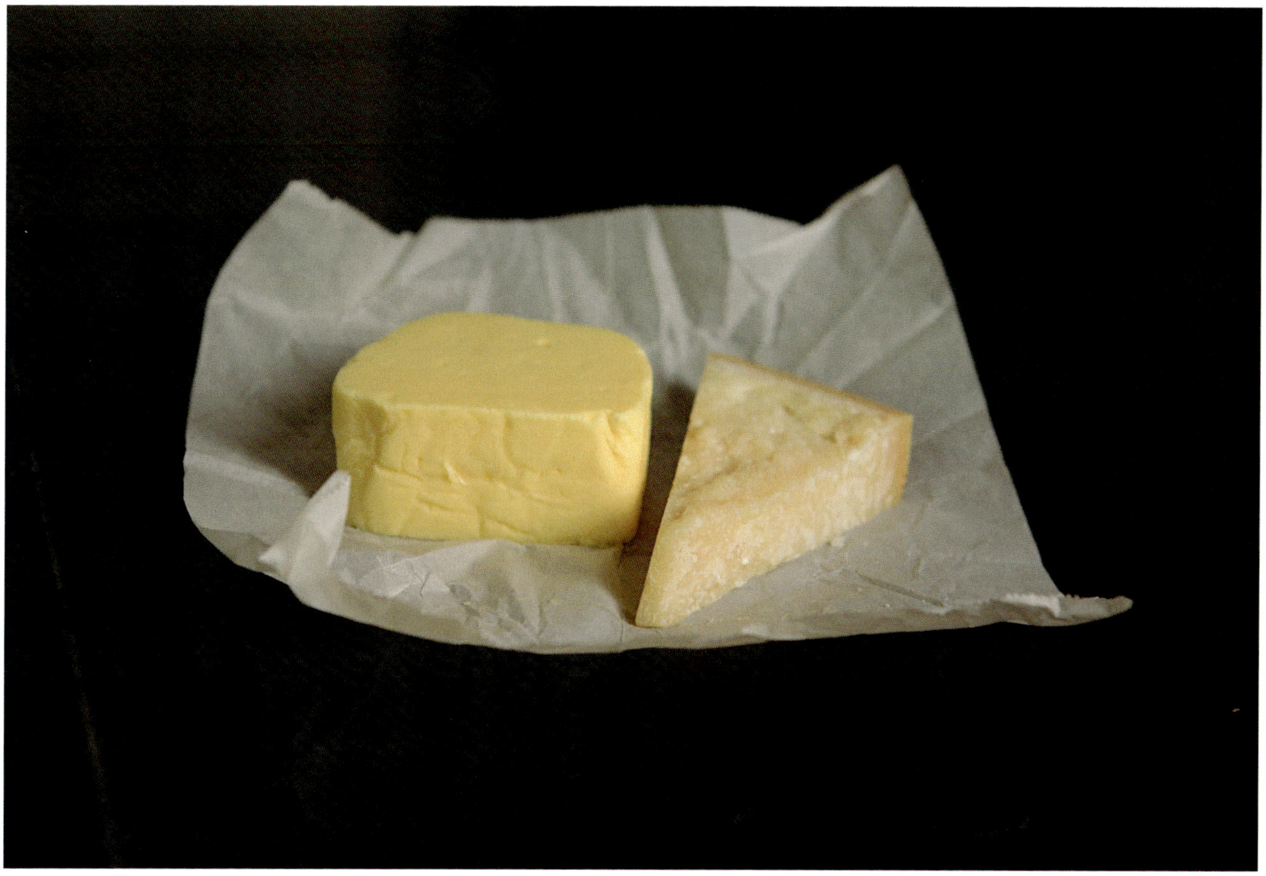

If you are prone to firm bowel movements or constipation: Eat more high fat dairy like real sour cream (made from raw cream), crème fraîche, ghee, and butter. High protein dairy products such as yogurt, whey, kefir, and cheese may constipate you. Note: In severe cases of constipation, if you find that even eating large amounts of high fat dairy constipates, it may be a good idea to refrain from dairy until the constipation resolves and then begin slowly introducing it again.

If you are prone to diarrhea: Introduce homemade whey (see Making Whey from Raw Milk in chapter 7). Take 1 teaspoon per day for 1–5 days, then increase to 2 teaspoons per day, and so on. You will do better with yogurt and, eventually, cheese. These high protein dairy products will help "bind you," or firm up your bowels.

As always throughout this protocol, listen to your body. If you experience constipation when you introduce yogurt, eat less yogurt and more crème fraîche, raw sour cream, butter, and ghee. If you experience very loose bowel movements when you introduce crème fraîche and raw sour cream, eat them less, and eat yogurt more. That is the beauty and challenge of the Gut and Psychology Syndrome diet: you may (and must) tailor it to what your body needs.

General Digestibility Scale

High Fat: Easier to Digest → **High Protein: Hard to Digest**

Ghee — Butter — Crème Fraîche — Kefir from Cream — Yogurt or Kefir from Milk — Hard Cheeses

Culturing Dairy

The Recipes

7

Now that you have an idea of what cultured dairy is, as well as how and when to introduce it into your diet, you can move on to the techniques for making the foods you will need to heal.

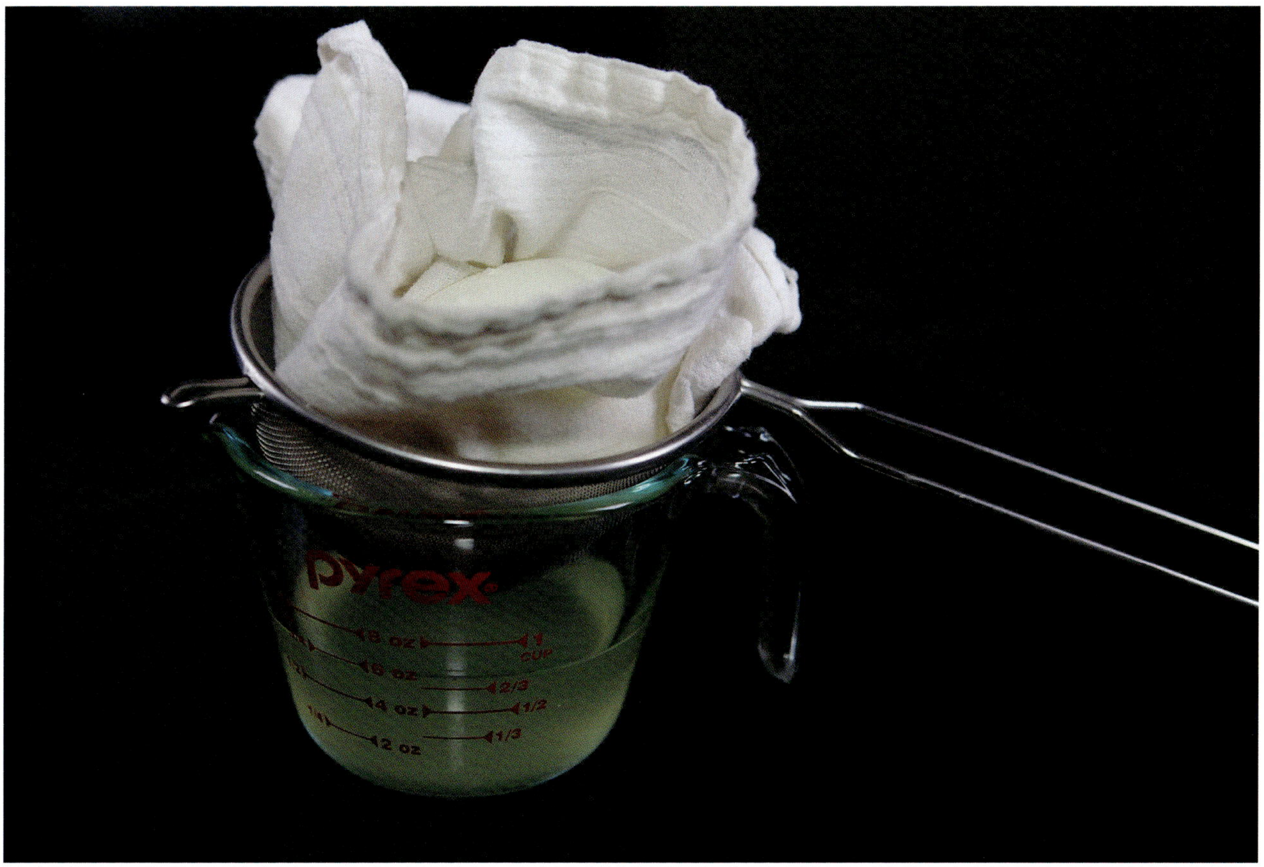

Before you get started, be sure to have the following equipment on hand:

Handy Kitchen Utensils for Culturing Dairy

- Wide-mouth quart jars with lids
- Wide-mouth pint jars with lids
- Cheesecloth, lint-free tea towels, or nut bags
- Canning funnel
- Instant read or digital thermometer
- Quart capacity thermos that will hold hot for 24 hours (this will be noted on label), yogurt maker, or dehydrator
- Small whisk to fit in jars
- 2-cup liquid measure, glass preferred
- Fine mesh strainer to fit in 2-cup liquid measure
- Full set of measuring spoons
- Flat wooden spoon
- Large stainless steel, ceramic, or glass bowl
- Food processor with S blade
- Small, fine plastic mesh strainer (for kefir)

Starters and Techniques

What is a starter? A "starter" is a bit of bacterial culture (or bacteria and yeast) that acts as an inoculant for milk or cream. You add some to your milk or cream to "start" the culturing process. Adding a starter helps load the deck in favor of beneficial microbes. You could say it gives them a head start!

Use a diversity of starters. Be creative in your culturing endeavors! The greater the diversity of starters you use, the more diverse bacteria you provide to your digestive system. There are many ways to culture milk in order to make yogurt, and there are many ways to culture cream in order to make crème fraîche, or cultured cream. Mix it up! Your digestive system—and your whole body—will thank you. You may heal more quickly, and your immune system will be more robust.

Whey

What is whey? Whey is a protein found in milk. It is a simple molecule, so your body absorbs it easily. Most people are not sensitive or allergic to whey. You can find it in powdered form at health food stores (sold as "whey protein powder"), but this is a highly processed product. The protein has most likely been denatured (i.e., damaged or restructured) by the processing. Whey powder is not permitted on the GAPS diet.

Homemade whey prepared from yogurt, kefir, or raw milk is best for this healing protocol. And as you will see below, it is very easy to make.

What is the role of whey in the GAPS diet? Whey has many roles in the GAPS diet. The most important is to provide your body with easily absorbed food-based probiotics from the start of the Intro diet. Whey contributes a valuable protein that is easily absorbed by the body. Whey can be used to inoculate or "start" culturing milk for yogurt or cream for crème fraîche. In addition, it will be used for the fermentation of vegetables, fruits, beverages, nuts, and seeds in later stages of the Intro diet. **When you graduate to the Full GAPS diet, you will use whey to ferment beans, and again when you transition off GAPS and are about to reintroduce grains into your diet.** The first grains you introduce will be fermented with whey. As you can see, it plays a very large role in the diet, so get jiggy with whey!

Important—do not make whey from pasteurized milk! Raw milk is the *only* milk you can safely leave at room temperature to separate into curds and whey. As noted previously, you should never attempt to make whey from pasteurized milk—it will make you very sick if you leave it on the counter at room temperature. Remember that pasteurization is sterilization: all of the protective bacteria you find in fresh, raw milk straight from the cow is destroyed by the pasteurizing process. What is left is a sterile environment where opportunistic, putrefying bacteria can multiply rapidly with no checks on their growth. This does not happen with raw milk as raw milk from grass-fed cows is chock-full of healthy bacteria (lactobacilli) that prevent the "bad guys" (the bacteria that makes you sick) from growing at room temperature.

Now let's learn the many ways you can make whey. These are foundational recipes, and you will be referring back to them in subsequent sections of this book.

Whey from Raw Milk

Yields about 1 cup yogurt cheese and 3 cups whey.

Ingredients

½ gallon raw milk (do not use pasteurized milk)

Special equipment:
1 strainer, preferably cone-shaped, or nut milk bag
Cheesecloth, lint-free tea towel, or cotton napkin
2-cup liquid measure (to fit strainer) or bowl (to place under nut milk bag)

Instructions

1. To separate the curds from the whey, leave raw milk on the counter at room temperature, out of sunlight and tightly capped. In 3–5 days, the curds and whey will separate. The whey will be a lovely chartreuse-colored liquid on the bottom. The white or yellowish-white curds will be on top.

2. Strain. *If using nut milk bag:* No need for a strainer. Simply hang the filled nut milk bag over a bowl to catch the whey by either attaching it to a cabinet knob or using a large spoon to suspend the bag. *If using strainer:* Place strainer in liquid measure. Line with 2 layers of cheesecloth, tea towel, or napkin. Pour the separated raw milk (the curds and whey from step 1) into strainer. The whey will drip into the liquid measure, and the cheese will remain in the cheesecloth.

3. Leave on counter to strain 12–36 hours. The longer you drip, the firmer the cheese. Store whey and cheese in tightly closed glass jars in the refrigerator. Whey will last in the refrigerator for up to 6 months.

Note: The milk solids will be creamy if eaten right away, with a texture like cream cheese. You may also allow the solids to strain longer. The cheese will become firmer the longer you allow the whey to drip from it.

Whey from Yogurt: "Dripping or Straining Whey" Technique

It is best to use homemade yogurt here (see Chapter 7: The Recipes). When necessary, you may purchase commercial yogurt without fillers or additives. However, be sure to use organic, plain, whole milk yogurt from grass-fed cows whenever possible. If you do use homemade yogurt, it may be very runny—much more so than commercial yogurt—so you may need to use several layers of cheesecloth in order to cleanly separate the solids from the whey. A tea towel or linen napkin may prove easier to use.

One quart of yogurt will yield approximately 2 cups of whey and 1 cup of yogurt cheese.

Ingredients

1 quart good-quality, plain, organic, whole-milk yogurt (no fillers, from pastured cows if possible, homemade is best)

Special equipment:
1 strainer (preferably cone-shaped) or nut milk bag
Cheesecloth, lint-free tea towel, or cotton napkin
2-cup liquid measure (to fit strainer) or bowl (to place under nut milk bag)

Instructions

1. Strain. *If using nut milk bag:* No need for a strainer. Simply hang the filled nut milk bag over a bowl to catch the whey by either attaching it to a cabinet knob or using a large spoon to suspend the bag. *If using strainer:* Place strainer in liquid measure. Line with a few layers of cheesecloth, tea towel, or napkin. Spoon yogurt into strainer. The whey will drip into the liquid measure, and the yogurt cheese will remain in the cheesecloth.
2. Leave on counter 12–36 hours. The longer you drip, the firmer the cheese.
3. Store the whey and the cheese in separate glass jars in the refrigerator. Whey will last in the refrigerator for up to 6 months.

What Is Yogurt Cheese or Kefir Cheese? What Can You Do with It?

The soft, creamy cheese left in the lined strainer or nut milk bag is yogurt cheese or kefir cheese, depending upon which one you dripped to make the whey. It is similar to commercial cream cheese but so much better for you. This cheese has live enzymes and good bacteria for your digestive system, and it does not contain fillers! As you get further along on the Intro diet, you can make the yogurt or kefir cheese sweet (by adding in a touch of honey) or savory (by adding in such ingredients as fresh herbs and garlic).

Whey from Kefir: "Dripping or Straining Whey" Technique

When making whey from kefir, homemade kefir is best. When necessary, you may use commercial brands without fillers or additives. If you choose to purchase kefir, make sure it is organic, plain, whole milk kefir. Due to its consistency, tea towels, napkins, or nut milk bags work best for this process. Kefir tends to be runny and will not easily separate with cheesecloth. (Using a cheesecloth to strain kefir will not yield a clean, pure kefir whey. The milk solids seep through the cheesecloth unless you use several layers, as with the homemade yogurt above.)

Yields 2 cups whey and 1 cup kefir cheese.

Ingredients

1 quart good-quality, plain, organic, whole-milk kefir (no fillers, from pastured cows if possible, homemade is best)

Special equipment:
1 strainer, preferably cone-shaped, or nut milk bag
Cheesecloth, lint-free tea towel, or cotton napkin
2-cup liquid measure (to fit strainer) or bowl (to place under nut milk bag)

Instructions

1. Strain. *If using nut milk bag:* No need for a strainer. Simply hang the filled nut milk bag over a bowl to catch the whey by either attaching it to a cabinet knob or using a large spoon to suspend the bag. *If using strainer:* Place strainer in liquid measure. Line with a few layers of cheesecloth, tea towel, or napkin. Spoon kefir into strainer. The whey will drip into the liquid measure, and the kefir cheese will remain in the cheesecloth.

2. Leave on counter to strain 12–36 hours. The longer you drip, the firmer the cheese.

3. Store whey and cheese in tightly closed glass jars in the refrigerator. Whey will last in the refrigerator for up to 6 months.

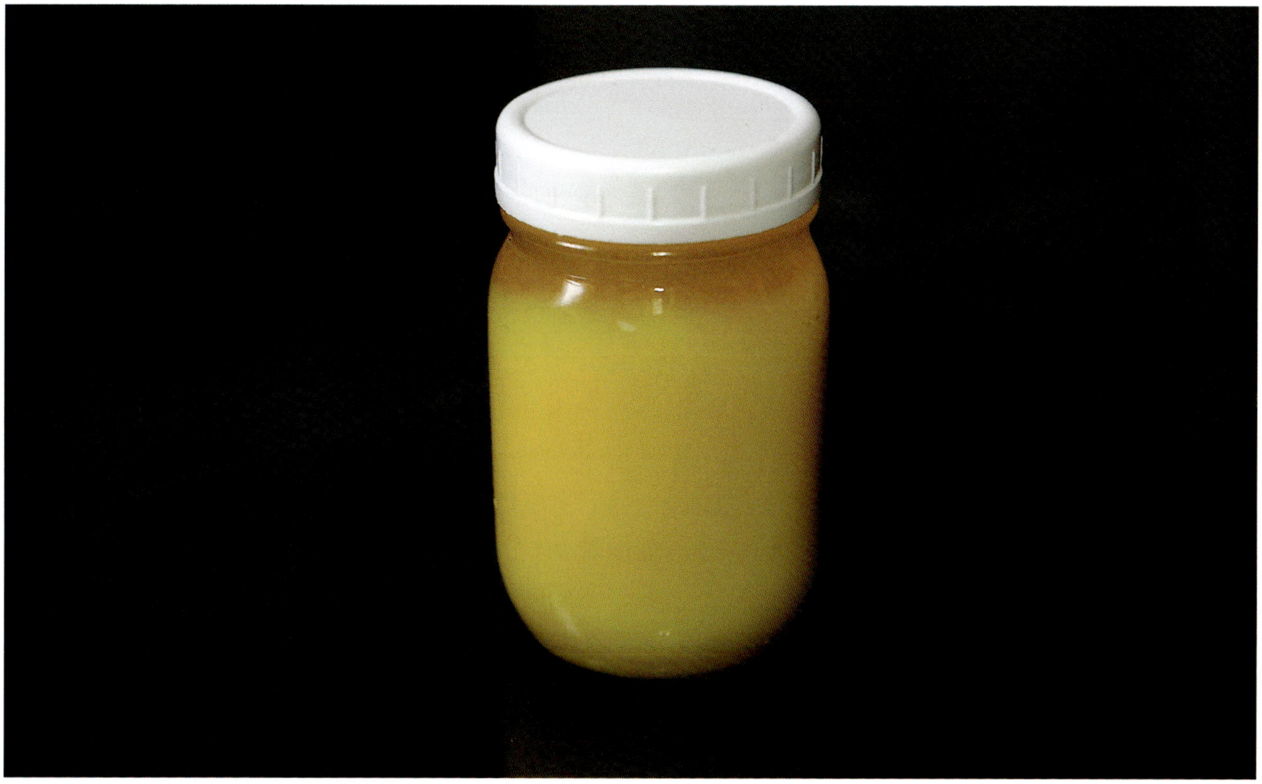

Ghee

What is ghee? Ghee is clarified butter with all of the milk solids removed, leaving pure fat. Because ghee is pure fat with no milk solids, it does not contain lactose or casein, both of which are problematic to a damaged digestive system. As pure fat, ghee is the easiest to digest. Almost everyone can tolerate it, even those with dairy allergies or sensitivities.

What is the role of ghee in the GAPS diet? Ghee is used liberally throughout the GAPS Intro diet. It is also introduced first in the Dairy Introduction Protocol (see chapter 5) because it is the easiest dairy product for most people to tolerate.

It is important to consume a large amount of healthy fats when on the GAPS Diet, and ghee is one of them. Feel free to add a tablespoon or more of ghee to every mug of Meat Stock, soup, or stew prior to consuming. Later you will use ghee to sauté vegetables and adorn those sautéed vegetables prior to serving. When you are on the Full GAPS Diet, you will use ghee to make healthy, delicious treats.

Making Ghee

The greater amount of butter you use, the easier it is to make ghee. So double or triple the following recipe if you can.

Ingredients

1 lb. or more of pastured butter

Instructions

1. Preheat oven to 140–250°F. Place butter in a pan and slowly melt in the oven. Alternatively, you may heat butter in a saucepot on the stove at very low temperature.
2. In 30–60 minutes, butter will separate into 3 layers: a white foamy crust on top, liquid gold in the middle, and white milk solids on the bottom. Watch your ghee carefully. The amount of time it will take to melt will be directly related to the temperature of your oven or stove. You do not want to boil the ghee!
3. Remove the solids on top with a spoon, without disturbing the milk solids on the bottom. Milk solids will look like milk. They will not be "solid."
4. Ladle off the liquid gold into a jar. (You may wish to strain it through several layers of cheesecloth or a linen towel and strainer to be sure that no milk solids remain.)
5. When you get to the bottom of the pan and it becomes difficult to separate the liquid from the solids, place the pan in the refrigerator to cool completely. When cooled, pour off the liquid—milk solids—and pop off the ghee.

Note: Ghee may be stored at room temperature, so no need to refrigerate.

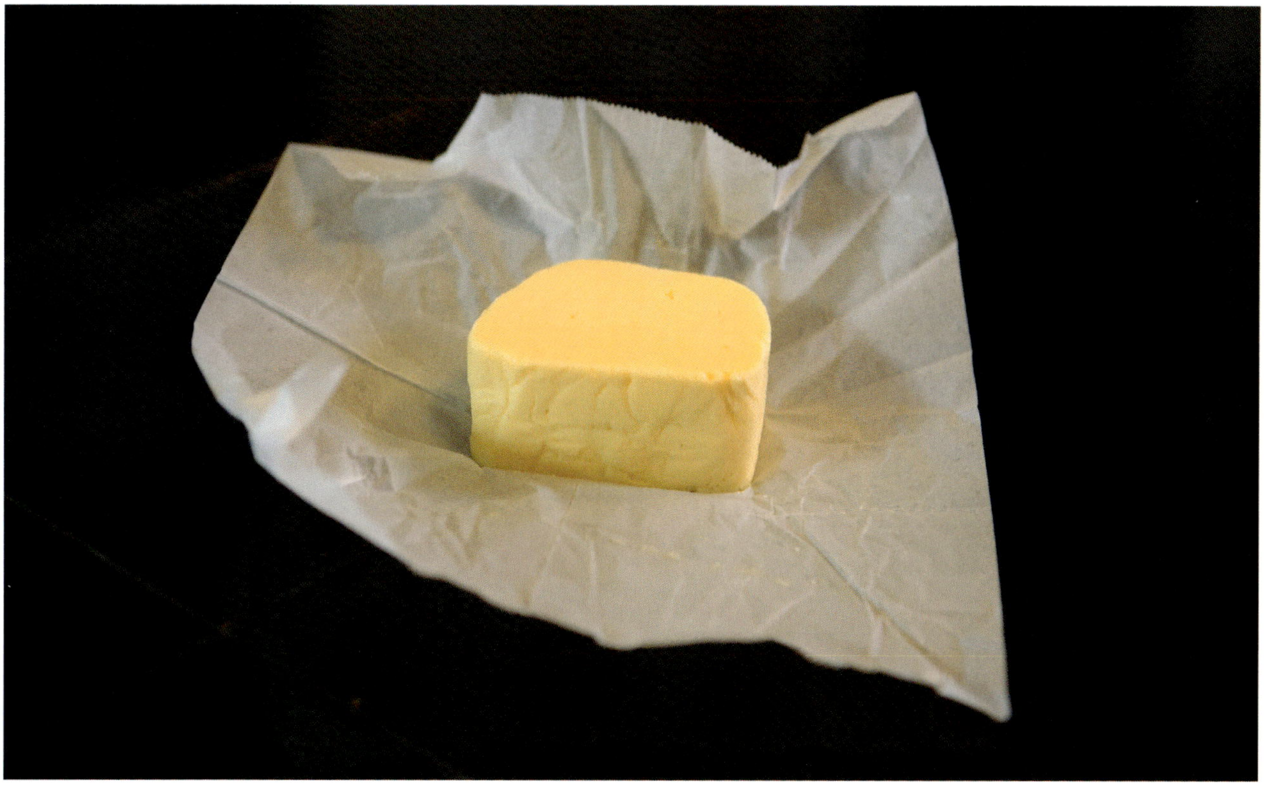

Cultured Butter

What is cultured butter? Cultured butter is butter made from cream that has been cultured. You know by now that "cream that has been cultured" is crème fraîche. Make your own first (see the crème fraîche recipes in this chapter) or purchase commercially available crème fraîche that lists *only* cream and cultures in the ingredients. No fillers allowed. Also, in order to be sure that all of the lactose is predigested, keep your store-bought crème fraîche on the counter for 24 hours, then proceed to make it into butter.

What is the role of cultured butter in the GAPS diet? Cultured butter is used liberally throughout the Intro diet and the Full GAPS diet as it is a healthy fat that is easily digested by the body. For those doing the Dairy Introduction Protocol, it is the second food introduced to the diet. Butter itself is mostly fat, with some whey. To make the butter, use crème fraîche that has been cultured a minimum 24 hours to ensure it is also lactose-free.

Making Cultured Butter

Ingredients

1 quart or more homemade crème fraîche (preferred), or commercially prepared organic crème fraîche with no fillers, cultured an additional 24 hours in a glass jar on the counter

Instructions

1. Pour the crème fraîche into a food processor that is fitted with an S blade. Process until a ball of butter forms along with buttermilk. (Buttermilk is the liquid that separates from the fat—which is butter!) Alternatively, use a glass jar or churn to separate the butter from the buttermilk, keeping in mind that this will take much more time than a food processor.

2. Remove the ball of butter. Place in a large bowl. Press the ball against the sides of the bowl with a flat wooden spoon to press out more buttermilk.

3. Carefully pour the buttermilk into a jar and reserve. You may wish to pour through a strainer lined with cheesecloth in order to catch any stray butter bits.

4. Pat the butter dry with a towel. Store in a butter bell, crock, or jar in the refrigerator. Alternatively, if you prefer soft, spreadable butter, store on the counter at room temperature. You may also store butter in the freezer in an airtight container if you make a large batch.

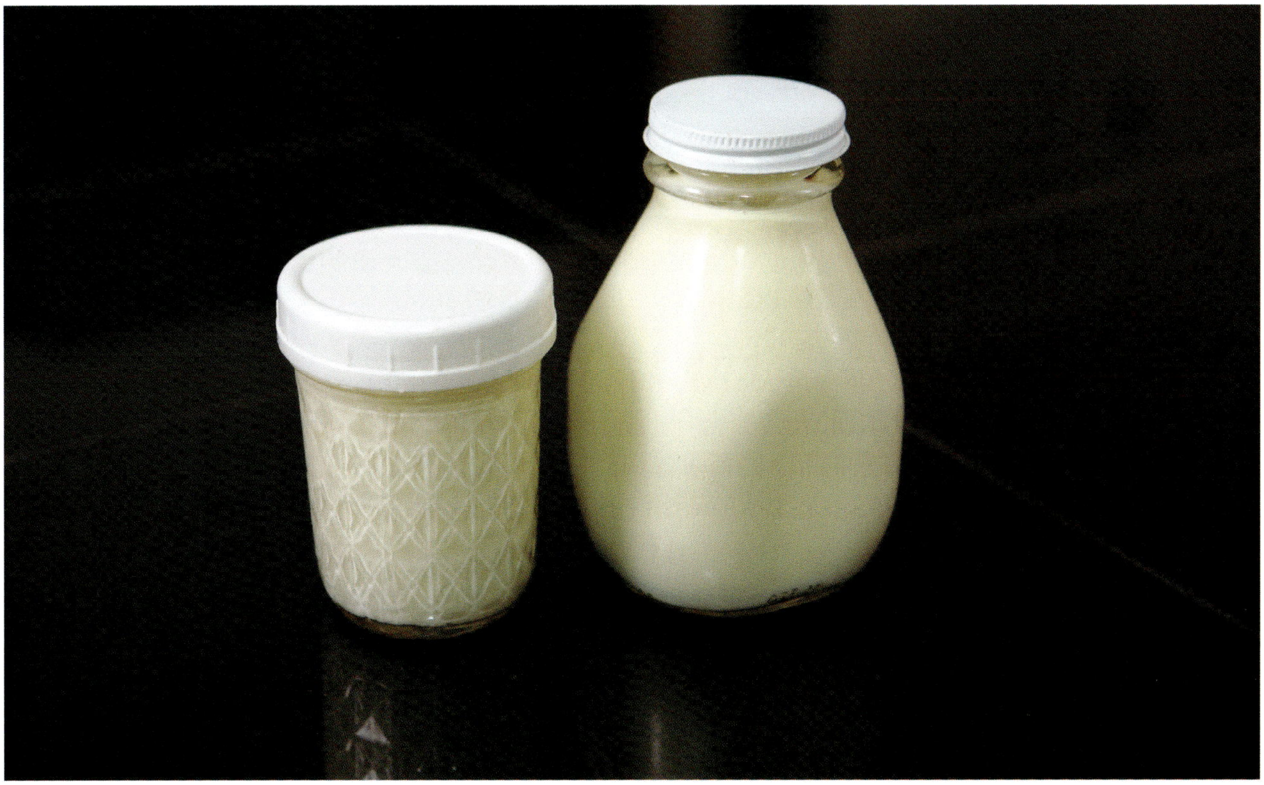

Crème Fraîche (Cultured Cream)

What is crème fraîche? Crème fraîche is cream that has been cultured. It is very rich in good fat, enzymes, and probiotics. Crème fraîche is also considered a high fat dairy product, which means it is especially good for people on this healing protocol. Remember, individuals with damaged guts need a lot of healthy saturated fats. Note: Crème fraîche will firm up in the refrigerator over time.

If you are prone to constipation, eat high fat dairy such as crème fraîche to keep things moving. On the other hand, avoid high *protein* dairy such as yogurt, which will constipate those who are prone to constipation.

Making Crème Fraîche from Whey

The flavor of crème fraîche depends on the type of whey you choose. As stated previously, the whey you obtain from dripping yogurt or kefir has a different profile of bacteria, or bacteria and yeast cultures, than whey you obtain by allowing *raw* milk to separate on the counter. Each batch has different types of bacteria or yeast (or bacteria and yeast in the case of whey dripped from kefir) that will grow in your cream and culture it. Depending on the different bacteria and yeast you use, each method will yield a different flavor and texture in the final product. This is a good thing.

Note: The longer you culture the cream, the more sour it will become. This is normal. The good bacteria (or good bacteria and yeast) eat all the milk sugar (lactose), which is responsible for making the cream or milk sweet. We do not want sweet—we want predigested (sour).

Ingredients

1 pint raw cream or organic heavy cream from grass-fed cows (pasteurized okay, but not UHT)
¼ cup whey from yogurt, kefir, or raw milk

Instructions

1. Pour cream into a small saucepot. Gently heat on the stove at low temperature. Use a thermometer (digital is easiest) to bring cream to 100–110°F. If you are using pasteurized cream, bring it to 180°F, then let it cool down to 100–110°F before culturing. Raw cream does not need to be heated at all, but if you prefer a firmer product, you could heat it only to 100–110°F.
2. Pour cream into a pint-sized wide-mouth glass jar.
3. Add whey and stir together to mix well. Cap the jar and leave on the counter for a minimum of 24 hours.
4. Refrigerate and consume liberally!

Making Crème Fraîche from Crème Fraîche

Ingredients

1 pint raw cream or organic heavy cream from grass-fed cows (pasteurized okay, but not UHT)
¼ cup crème fraîche (store-bought or from a previous batch)

Instructions

1. Pour cream into a small saucepot. Gently heat on the stove at low temperature. Use a thermometer (digital is easiest) to bring cream to 100–110°F. If you are using pasteurized cream, bring it to 180°F, then let it cool down to 100–110°F before culturing. Raw cream does not need to be heated at all, but if you prefer a firmer product, you could heat it only to 100–110°F.
2. Pour cream into a pint-sized wide-mouth glass jar.
3. Add crème fraîche and stir together to mix well. Cap the jar and leave on the counter for a minimum of 24 hours.
4. Refrigerate and consume liberally!

Making Crème Fraîche from Yogurt

Ingredients

1 pint raw cream or organic heavy cream from grass-fed cows (pasteurized okay, but not UHT)
¼ cup homemade yogurt (preferred), or commercially prepared organic, plain, whole milk yogurt with no fillers

Instructions

1. Pour cream into a small saucepot. Gently heat on the stove at low temperature. Use a thermometer (digital is easiest) to bring the cream to 100–110°F. If you are using pasteurized cream, bring it to 180°F, then let it cool down to 100–110°F before culturing. Raw cream does not need to be heated at all, but if you prefer a firmer product, you could heat it only to 100–110°F.
2. Pour cream into a pint-sized wide-mouth glass jar.
3. Add yogurt and stir together to mix well. Cap the jar and leave on the counter for a minimum of 24 hours.
4. Refrigerate and consume liberally!

Commercial Grade Crème Fraîche Shortcut

If you are traveling or cannot make your own crème fraîche for some other reason, here is a shortcut that works: Purchase the best quality plain, organic, whole milk crème fraîche you can find. Make sure it does not contain any fillers. The best commercial crème fraîche will list only the following ingredients on the label: organic cream and bacterial cultures. Leave the crème fraîche out on the counter for 24 hours or more at room temperature. This ensures the lactose is predigested before you eat it. Remember, commercially produced crème fraîche is not cultured long enough to predigest the lactose. If the store-bought crème fraîche is in a plastic container, it is also a good idea to transfer it to a glass jar prior to leaving it on the counter. After 24 hours, place the crème fraîche in the refrigerator.

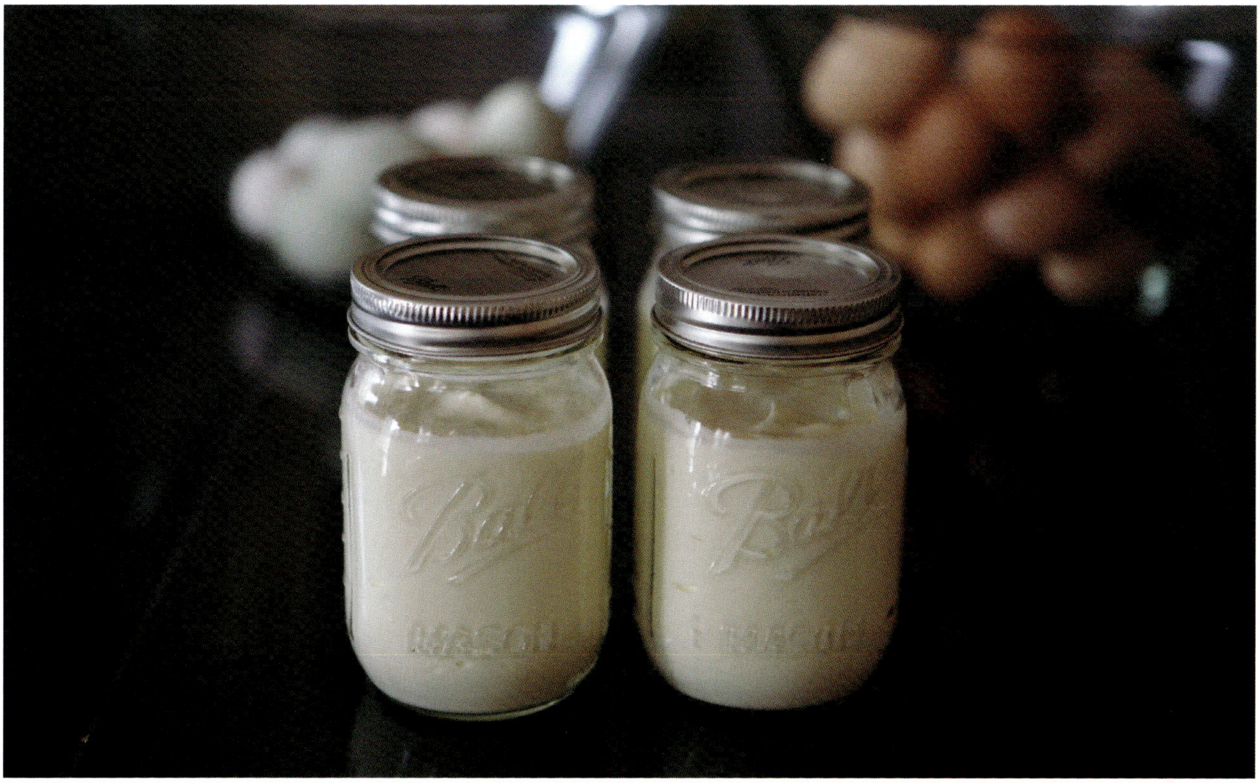

Yogurt

What is yogurt? Yogurt is milk that has been cultured. Lactic acid-producing bacteria, or lactobacilli, are added to the milk and encouraged to grow by eating all of the milk sugar (that is, predigesting the lactose). Yogurt may be drinkable, strained, or some consistency in between.

Why make your own yogurt? Store-bought yogurt can be fraught with problems for everyone, but it can especially be a problem for those on the GAPS diet. The milk may be low quality or have a low fat content, and it may contain fillers such as pectin and guar gum. Even some organic producers add fillers. Remember, GAPS is a *healing* diet. It is important to use the best quality ingredients you can find to ensure the quality of the yogurt you eat. Even if you find plain yogurt made from grass-fed, organic, whole milk with no fillers, it still will not be of any benefit because commercially available yogurt has not been cultured long enough to guarantee the therapeutic result we want. Most store-bought yogurt has been cultured only long enough to culture the milk but not long enough to predigest the lactose.

The key to making therapeutic-grade yogurt fit for the GAPS diet: You can make yogurt many ways. Once you obtain the best milk you can find, the next most important part is to make sure the lactose is predigested in the process. This is directly related to the amount of time you culture the milk and the temperature at which you culture it. To make lactose-free yogurt for the GAPS diet, you must culture milk for a minimum of 24 hours at 110°F.

Temperatures for Culturing Milk

The temperature you heat your milk prior to culturing depends on whether or not the milk is raw or pasteurized. Heat *raw milk* to 110°F, then add the culture or starter. Heat *pasteurized milk* to 180°F to kill any pathogenic bacteria that may have grown after the milk was pasteurized (sterilized). Once it has reached 180°F, cool it to 110°F prior to adding the culture or starter. Lowering the temperature to 110°F ensures that the bacteria necessary to culture the milk will not be killed off by high heat.

Techniques for making yogurt: For the following recipes, you may use a yogurt maker, thermos, electric plate, dehydrator, or a gas oven with a pilot light. Whichever technique you choose, the key is to hold the milk at 110°F for a minimum of 24 hours. If you use a jar or thermos, you must also be sure to keep the lid on. For all methods *except* the yogurt maker, you need to heat the milk on the stove beforehand.

Do not destroy the enzymes in raw milk! If you heat raw milk too high, you will destroy the live enzymes and good bacteria. Heat to 110°F and culture.

How to cool pasteurized milk rapidly for yogurt making: As stated, you must first heat pasteurized milk to 180°F, then cool it down to 110°F prior to adding the culture. One way to do this quickly is to fill your sink or a large bowl with ice and place the entire pot into the ice bath. Stir the milk while the pot rests in the ice; it will cool more quickly than if you just leave it on the stove. Take care to watch the temperature while cooling so it does not drop below 110°F—or you will be back to the stove to heat it up again!

Making Yogurt from Whey

Ingredients

1 quart raw milk, or organic milk from grass-fed cows (pasteurized okay, but not UHT)
⅓ cup whey from yogurt, kefir, or raw milk

Instructions

Yogurt maker:

1. Whisk ingredients together well.
2. Place in yogurt maker for a minimum of 24 hours.
3. When done, pour into glass jar and refrigerate.

Thermos:

1. Heat raw milk to 110°F. Alternatively, heat pasteurized milk to 180°F, then cool to 110°F.
2. Pour whey into the thermos. When the temperature of the milk is 110°F, add it to the thermos. Cap tightly, and hold at 110°F for a minimum of 24 hours. When done, place in refrigerator.

Electric plate, dehydrator, or gas oven with pilot light:

1. Heat raw milk to 110°F. Alternatively, heat pasteurized milk to 180°F, then cool to 110°F.
2. Pour whey into a glass jar. When the temperature of the milk is 110°F, add it to the jar. Place on the electric plate, or on the bottom of your dehydrator with the shelves removed. If your oven has a pilot light that holds the temperature at 110°F, place the jar on a sheet pan on the bottom shelf. Hold the jar at 110°F for a minimum of 24 hours. When done, place in refrigerator.

Making Yogurt from Yogurt

Ingredients

1 quart raw milk, or organic milk from grass-fed cows (pasteurized okay, but not UHT)
⅓ cup yogurt, store-bought or previous batch

Instructions

Yogurt maker:

1. Whisk ingredients together well.
2. Place in yogurt maker for a minimum of 24 hours.
3. When done, pour into glass jar and refrigerate.

Thermos:

1. Heat raw milk to 110°F. Alternatively, heat pasteurized milk to 180°F, then cool to 110°F.
2. Pour yogurt into the thermos. When the temperature of the milk is 110°F, add it to the thermos. Cap tightly, and hold at 110°F for a minimum of 24 hours. When done, place in refrigerator.

Electric plate, dehydrator, or gas oven with pilot light:

1. Heat raw milk to 110°F. Alternatively, heat pasteurized milk to 180°F, then cool to 110°F.
2. Pour yogurt into a glass jar. When the temperature of the milk is 110°F, add it to the jar. Place on the electric plate, or on the bottom of your dehydrator with the shelves removed. If your oven has a pilot light that holds the temperature at 110°F, place the jar on a sheet pan on the bottom shelf. Hold the jar at 110°F for a minimum of 24 hours. When done, place in refrigerator.

Making Yogurt from Crème Fraîche

Ingredients

1 quart raw milk, or organic milk from grass-fed cows (pasteurized okay, but not UHT)
⅓ cup crème fraîche, store-bought or previous batch

Instructions

Yogurt maker:

1. Whisk ingredients together well.
2. Place in yogurt maker for a minimum of 24 hours.
3. When done, pour into glass jar and refrigerate.

Thermos:

1. Heat raw milk to 110°F. Alternatively, heat pasteurized milk to 180°F, then cool to 110°F.
2. Pour crème fraîche into the thermos. When the temperature of the milk is 110°F, add it to the thermos. Cap tightly, and hold at 110°F for a minimum of 24 hours. When done, place in refrigerator.

Electric plate, dehydrator, or gas oven with pilot light:

1. Heat raw milk to 110°F. Alternatively, heat pasteurized milk to 180°F, then cool to 110°F.
2. Pour crème fraîche into a glass jar. When the temperature of the milk is 110°F, add it to the jar. Place on the electric plate, or on the bottom of your dehydrator with the shelves removed. If your oven has a pilot light that holds the temperature at 110°F, place the jar on a sheet pan on the bottom shelf. Hold the jar at 110°F for a minimum of 24 hours. When done, place in refrigerator.

Making Yogurt from Starter

Ingredients

1 quart raw milk, or organic milk from grass-fed cows (pasteurized okay, but not UHT)
1 yogurt starter packet

Instructions

Yogurt maker:

1. Whisk ingredients together well.
2. Place in yogurt maker for a minimum of 24 hours.
3. When done, pour into glass jar and refrigerate.

Thermos:

1. Heat raw milk to 110°F. Alternatively, heat pasteurized milk to 180°F, then cool to 110°F.
2. Pour starter into the thermos. When the temperature of the milk is 110°F, add it to the thermos. Cap tightly, and hold at 110°F for a minimum of 24 hours. When done, place in refrigerator.

Electric plate, dehydrator, or gas oven with pilot light:

1. Heat raw milk to 110°F. Alternatively, heat pasteurized milk to 180°F, then cool to 110°F.
2. Pour starter into a glass jar. When the temperature of the milk is 110°F, add it to the jar. Place on the electric plate, or on the bottom of your dehydrator with the shelves removed. If your oven has a pilot light that holds the temperature at 110°F, place the jar on a sheet pan on the bottom shelf. Hold the jar at 110°F for a minimum of 24 hours. When done, place in refrigerator.

What If Your Yogurt Is Too Runny or Not Thick Enough?

Homemade yogurt from raw milk often has a runnier, more liquid consistency than what you are used to seeing in commercially produced yogurt. If this is the case, simply strain some of the whey out of the yogurt to attain your preferred consistency. You can store the whey in a glass jar in the refrigerator for up to 6 months. You may use it as an inoculant or starter for yogurt or crème fraîche or as probiotic juice for Meat Stock or soups in the Intro diet.

Commercial Grade Yogurt Shortcut

If you are traveling or cannot make your own yogurt for some other reason, here is a shortcut that works: Purchase the best quality plain, organic, whole milk yogurt you can find. Make sure it does not contain any fillers. Leave the yogurt out on the counter for 24 hours or more. This ensures the lactose is predigested before you eat it. Remember, commercially produced yogurt is not cultured long enough to predigest the lactose. If the store-bought yogurt is in a plastic container, it is also a good idea to transfer it to a glass jar prior to leaving it on the counter. After 24 hours, place the yogurt in the refrigerator.

Mesophilic Yogurt—Almost as Easy to Make as Kefir

What is mesophilic yogurt? Mesophilic yogurt is yogurt that cultures at room temperature. Though it is not specific to the GAPS diet, mesophilic yogurt is so simple to make—and it includes other varieties of lactobacilli—that I thought I should include it here. It just may make your life a little easier.

Unlike all of the yogurt techniques above, making mesophilic yogurt requires the purchase of a starter culture. Visit Culturesforhealth.com for a mesophilic yogurt starter such as Viili, which has cultures that originate from Finland.

Making "Greek Style" Yogurt

"Greek" yogurt has become very popular in recent years. Originally, it was made with cultures specific to Greece that were not used in American yogurts. Now Greek yogurt is merely yogurt that has been strained of whey. You can make your own Greek-style yogurt simply by straining the whey from the yogurt until you achieve the desired consistency.

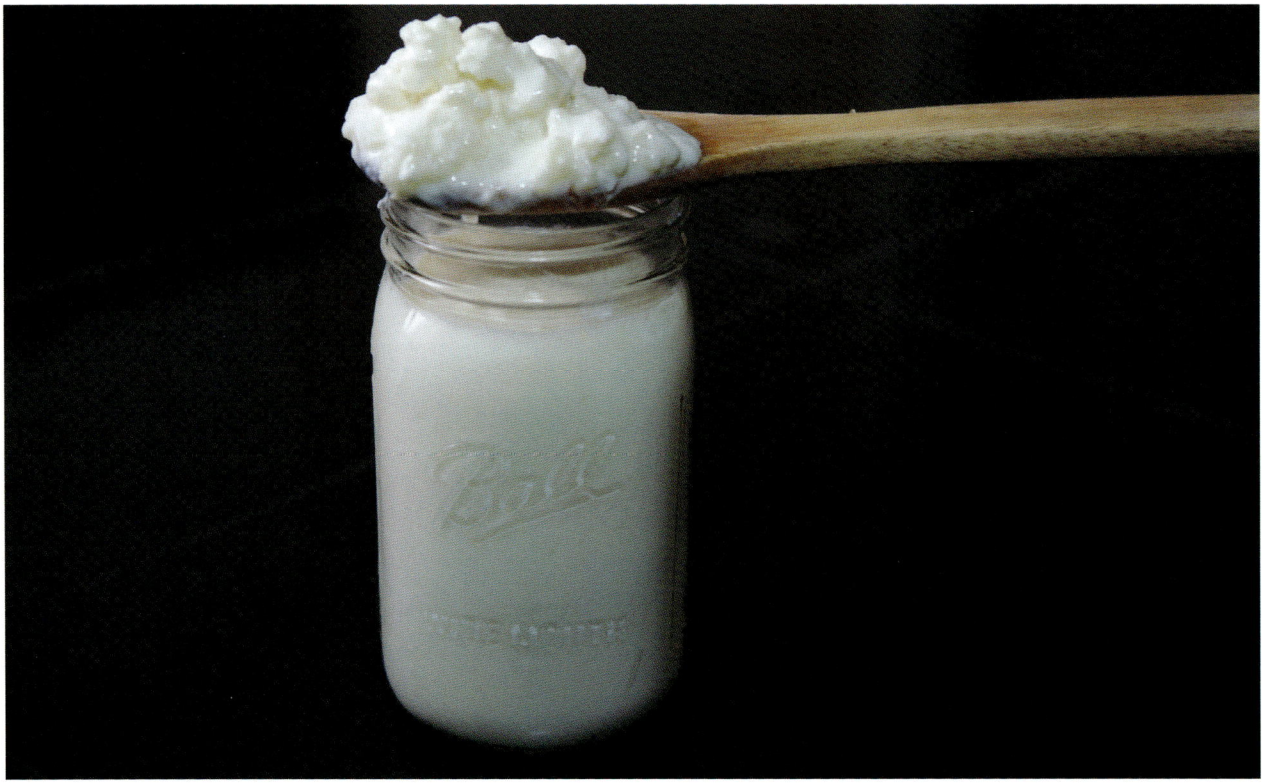

Kefir

What is kefir? Kefir is cultured milk that originated in the North Caucasus Mountains. A combination of bacteria and yeast is used to culture the milk and break down the lactose. Kefir is rich in healing lactic acid. You do not have to heat the milk or cream to make kefir. Also, many people think it is easier to make kefir than yogurt because there is no need to heat the milk first, and there are fewer steps.

Introduce kefir made from cream into your diet first. Once you can tolerate it, add kefir made from a combination of cream and milk to your diet, and finally add kefir made just from milk. As previously stated, higher fat dairy like cream is easier on your digestive system because it does not tend to cause constipation the way a high protein dairy like milk may.

Be cautious with kefir! Kefir is introduced last in the Dairy Introduction Protocol for a reason. You need to build up to introducing kefir to your diet because it can provoke a severe detoxification (detox) reaction if introduced too soon or in too great an amount. (Severe detox reactions can be flu-like symptoms, nausea, severe diarrhea or vomiting, or fever. They can also include brain fog, migraine headaches, eczema or skin flares, and mood swings, among other things.) Although kefir and yogurt are both cultured milk, they have different microbial profiles. Kefir contains yeast and bacterial cultures while yogurt contains only bacterial cultures. The yeast is the difference. So once again, slow and steady!

Making Kefir from Cream (with Kefir Grains)

Ingredients

1 quart raw cream, or organic heavy cream from grass-fed cows (pasteurized okay, but not UHT)
2 generous tablespoons kefir grains

Instructions

1. Stir together cream and grains in a wide-mouth glass jar. Cover loosely to allow oxygen in, which helps the yeast in the kefir grow.
2. Leave on the counter for a minimum of 24 hours.
3. Strain the grains out before drinking the kefir.
4. Start another batch, following the steps above.
5. Consume as desired.

How to store kefir grains: If you are not making kefir daily, refrigerate your grains in a glass jar with whole milk or cream, the best quality you can find, never UHT. Feed your grains fresh milk or cream once a week to keep them robust.

Making Kefir from Cream (with a Starter Packet)

Ingredients

1 quart raw cream, or organic heavy cream from grass-fed cows (pasteurized okay, but not UHT)
1 packet kefir starter

Instructions

1. Stir together cream and starter in a wide-mouth glass jar. Cover loosely to allow oxygen in, which helps the yeast in the kefir grow.
2. Leave on the counter for a minimum of 24 hours.
3. Retain ⅓ of the kefir to start the next batch.
4. Start another batch, following the steps in the next recipe, "Making Kefir from Cream (from a Previous Batch of Kefir)."
5. Consume as desired.

Making Kefir from Cream (from a Previous Batch of Kefir)

Ingredients

1 quart raw cream, or organic heavy cream from grass-fed cows (pasteurized okay, but not UHT)
⅓ cup kefir from a previous batch

Instructions

1. Stir together cream and kefir in a wide-mouth glass jar. Cover loosely to allow oxygen in, which helps the yeast in the kefir grow.
2. Leave on the counter for a minimum of 24 hours.
3. Retain ⅓ of the kefir to start the next batch.
4. Start another batch, following the steps above.
5. Consume as desired.

Making Kefir from Milk (with Kefir Grains)

Ingredients

1 quart raw milk, or organic whole milk from grass-fed cows (pasteurized okay, but not UHT)
2 generous tablespoons kefir grains

Instructions

1. Stir together milk and grains in a wide-mouth glass jar. Cover loosely to allow oxygen in, which helps the yeast in the kefir grow.
2. Leave on the counter for a minimum of 24 hours.
3. Strain the grains out to drink the kefir.
4. Start another batch, following the steps above.
5. Consume as desired.

Making Kefir from Milk (with a Starter Packet)

Ingredients

1 quart raw milk, or organic whole milk from grass-fed cows (pasteurized okay, but not UHT)
1 packet kefir starter

Instructions

1. Stir together milk and starter in a wide-mouth glass jar. Cover loosely to allow oxygen in, which helps the yeast in the kefir grow.
2. Leave on the counter for a minimum of 24 hours.
3. Retain ⅓ of the kefir to start the next batch.
4. Start another batch, following the steps in the recipe below, "Making Kefir from Milk (from a Previous Batch of Kefir)."
5. Consume as desired.

Making Kefir from Milk (from a Previous Batch of Kefir)

Ingredients

1 quart raw milk, or organic whole milk from grass-fed cows (pasteurized okay, but not UHT)
⅓ cup kefir

Instructions

1. Stir together cream and kefir in a wide-mouth glass jar. Cover loosely to allow oxygen in, which helps the yeast in the kefir grow.
2. Leave on the counter for a minimum of 24 hours.
3. Retain ⅓ of the kefir to start the next batch.
4. Start another batch, following the steps above.
5. Consume as desired.

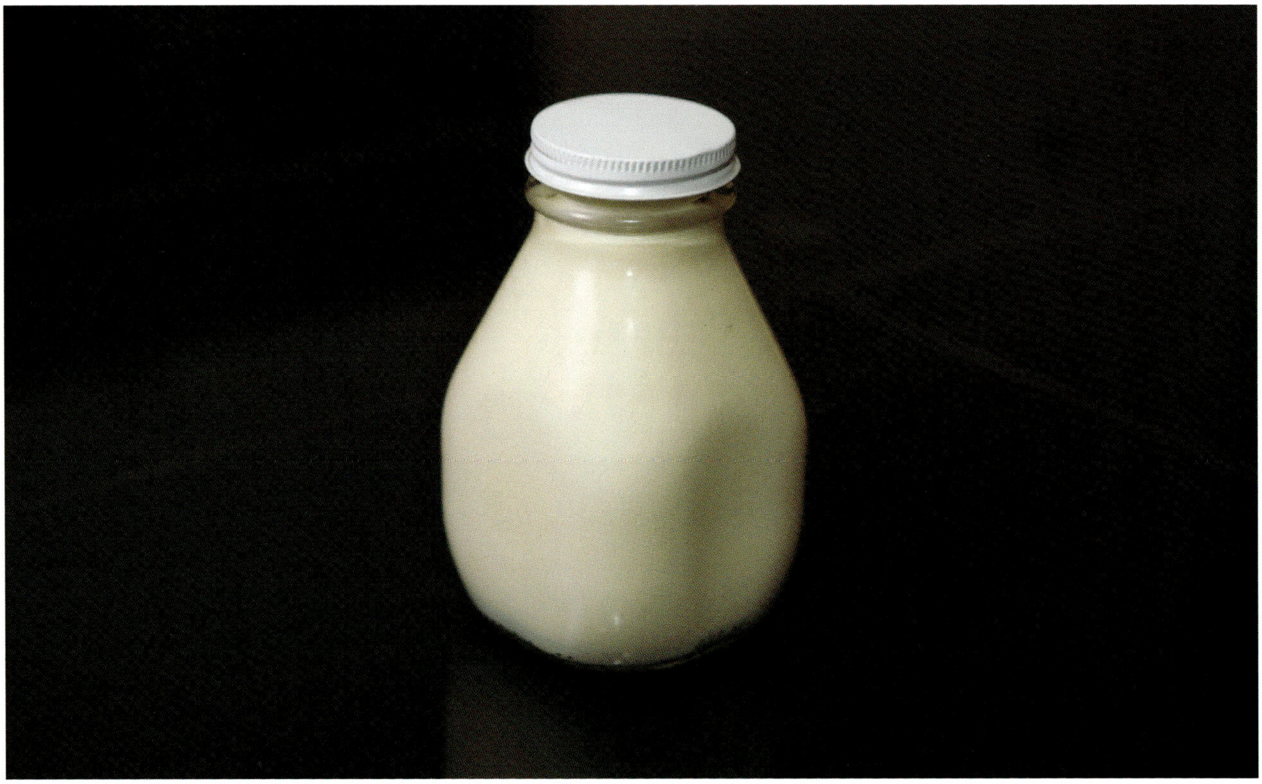

Sour Cream

What is sour cream? Sour cream is simply "soured cream," or cream that you allow to sour. As stated previously, sour cream must be made from *raw* cream. Raw cream sours over time because it is full of live bacteria that naturally consume all of the sweetness—that is, the milk sugar (lactose). As the bacteria consumes more and more lactose, the cream becomes more and more sour.

Why make sour cream? Sour cream is a cultured dairy product that is high in fat. Not only does it deliver enzymes, good bacteria, and lactic acid to the digestive tract, but it is also rich in fat-soluble vitamins A and D when made from cream from pastured cows. Because it is high fat, it will not constipate those who are prone to constipation. And it is delicious!

Remember to add sour cream to Meat Stock and soups only after they have cooled a bit, so as not to destroy the enzymes and bacteria.

Making Sour Cream from Raw Cream Only

It bears repeating—do *not* try this with pasteurized cream. It will putrefy and make you sick. Only raw cream will *sour*. Where can you find raw cream? If you are lucky enough to live in a state where you can purchase raw dairy from a certified farmer, you may be able to purchase raw cream directly from the farm. If not, you may skim the cream from the top of a jar of raw milk. The cream will come to the top of the jar of milk. You may skim the cream with a ladle. Once you skim the cream off the milk, you may use the milk for your garden! It is widely known among dairy farmers (the pastured dairy folks) that skimmed milk is only fit for fattening pigs. Skim milk is also used by biodynamic farmers on vegetable gardens because it's very good for crops. One would *never* drink skim milk. The body cannot use it.

Ingredients

Raw cream

Instructions

1. To make true sour cream, place raw cream in a glass jar and cover. Leave on the counter at room temperature for a minimum of 24 hours. However, 36 hours should guarantee that all of the lactose will be predigested for you.
2. After 24–36 hours, place the jar in the refrigerator.
3. The soured cream will be lactose free.
4. Consume liberally!

Note: It is a good idea to retain some of your sour cream (about a ¼ cup or so) to use as a starter for crème fraîche.

Culturing Dairy

Frequently Asked Questions

8

What is "healthy dairy"? Real milk comes from cows such as Guernseys and Jerseys raised on grass, hay, and root vegetables. Vital nutrients such as vitamins A and D are greatest in milk from grass-fed cows. In the United States, most milk, even organic, comes from cows that are not pastured. These cows live in confinement dairies and are fed grains (including genetically engineered soy and corn), cottonseed meal, and other feeds. Cows are not meant to eat grains. This kind of diet causes extreme gastric distress and sets up an environment of acidosis. Cows

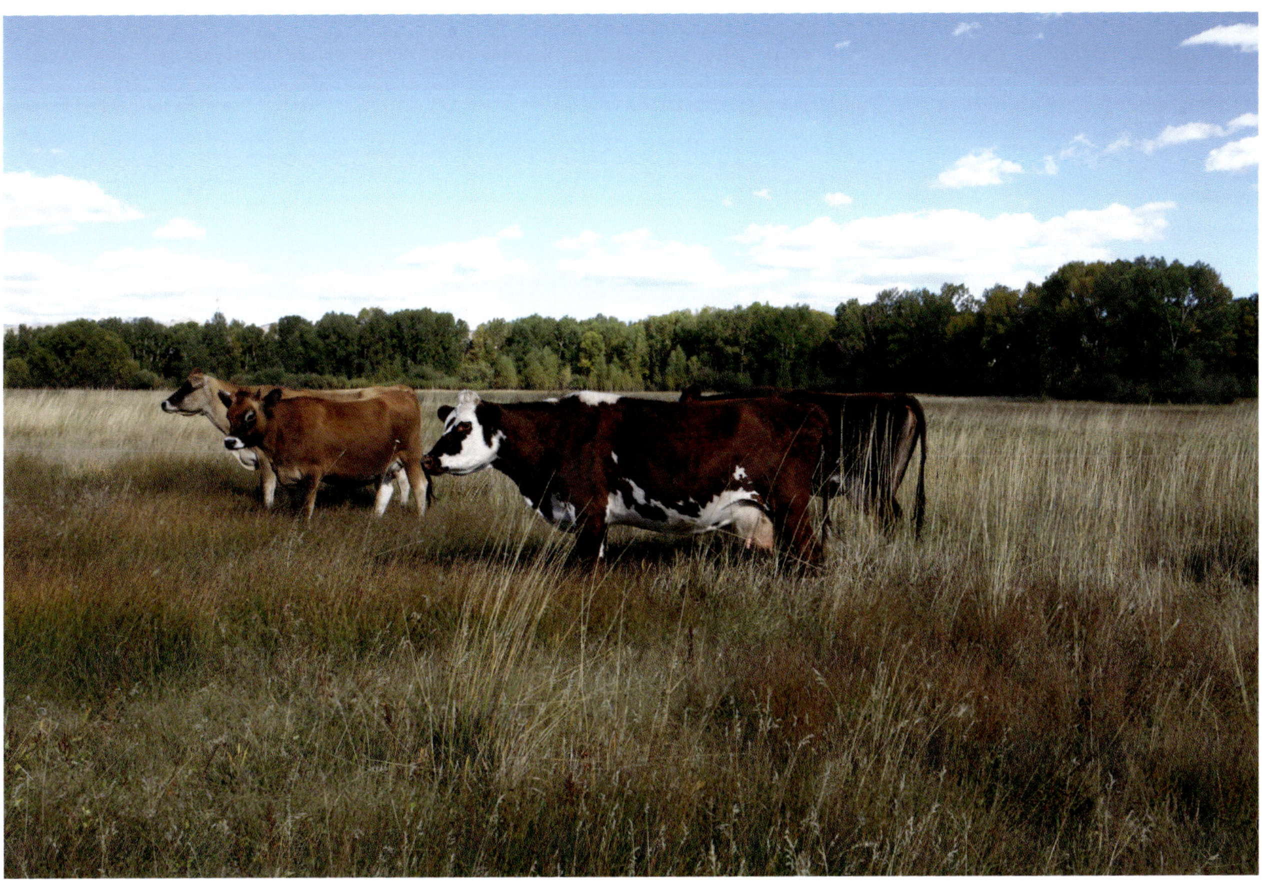

that are not pastured live half as long as pastured cows, according to Mark McAfee, founder and owner of Organic Pastures Dairy and founder of the Raw Milk Institute. (Read "Splendor from the Grass" by Sally Fallon and Mary G. Enig at WestonAPrice.org for more on the lifespan of pastured cows versus those in confinement.)

What is pasteurization? A process developed in 1864 by Louis Pasteur. In the 1880s in the United States, milk was pasteurized in order to sanitize milk that came from filthy confinement dairies in cities. When *real* milk sours, it becomes sour milk, which can be used in cooking and baking. When pasteurized milk sours, it becomes putrid and can make you sick.

Further, pasteurization is a process that:

- Destroys living enzymes
- Diminishes vitamin content, including vitamins C, B12, and B6
- Decreases the amount of calcium by approximately a third
- Denatures fragile proteins
- Kills beneficial bacteria
- Promotes the growth of opportunistic bacteria and pathogens

What is homogenization? This mechanical process breaks up the fats into tiny particles that do not rise to the top of the milk and create a cream line. Because of this, the fat in homogenized milk is more susceptible to rancidity and oxidation and will sour more quickly. In pasteurized milk, homogenization helps spread the dead white blood cells and bacteria throughout the milk. Not only is the cream evenly distributed, but the sludge is evenly distributed also. *Yuck.*

How does one store whey? It is best to store whey in a clean, tightly covered glass jar in the refrigerator. If you begin to see some white developing on the sides of the jar, simply wipe off the sides with a clean towel or paper towel and then transfer to a new jar.

How long will whey last in the refrigerator? Whey will last up to 6 months in the refrigerator when stored in a clean glass jar.

How do I know when to toss out my whey? Your nose knows. Whey should have a pleasing smell like yogurt. If whey begins to smell acrid or very sour, toss it. Make a new batch by straining yogurt or kefir or letting raw milk separate into curds and whey.

Which is better: cultured or raw butter? Culturing renders all dairy products easier to digest and contributes valuable enzymes, microbes, and vitamins. Culturing the cream you use to make butter for 24 hours or more will also predigest all of the lactose. Raw butter contains whey and some lactose, as it has not been predigested by culturing. As you know, enzymes are killed by heating. A good rule of thumb for the GAPS diet: if you are going to heat the butter, use *raw* butter. If you are going to eat the butter without heating or cooking it, use *cultured* butter!

Does refrigeration stop culturing? Yogurt, kefir, and crème fraîche will continue culturing in the refrigerator, albeit at a much slower pace than they would at room temperature. That means your cultured dairy products will get more sour the longer they remain in the refrigerator. So eat up sooner rather than later! (If these dairy products become "too sour" for your taste buds, you may use them later in the Intro diet and throughout the Full GAPS diet for baking with nuts and seeds. Never throw them out; they can also be used as a starter to culture your next batch or to marinate grass-fed meats.)

Should I invest in a digital or instant read thermometer? Yes! Digital and instant read thermometers are inexpensive and worth every penny! They make it very easy to be accurate when you are making yogurt.

Section IX | Lacto-Fermentation

Originally published in a single volume under the title *Cooking Techniques for the Gut and Psychology Syndrome™ Diet, Part III: Lacto-Fermentation*.

Foreword

> I would like to thank Monica Corrado for another wonderful resource for people who follow the GAPS nutritional protocol and for anybody who wants to introduce healthy foods into their diet! In this book she gives detailed explanations about how to make your own fermented foods at home.
>
> Many people don't realize that fermented foods are not optional for humans to consume. They are a must because for most of our existence on this planet we fermented a large part of the foods we consumed. Why? Because for much of that time, we didn't have refrigeration and supermarkets where we could buy any food out of its natural growing season. Foods were seasonal and difficult to obtain. When you worked hard in your garden and your cabbages were ripe in the autumn, you had to preserve them somehow because fresh cabbage will not keep for long.
>
> Fermentation—making sauerkraut—is an excellent way to preserve cabbage: it will keep well up to five years without spoiling! So, until next autumn our ancestors could consume cabbage in a fermented state, swallowing trillions of beneficial microbes and supporting our gut flora with every mouthful. Cabbage is just one example. In traditional societies all other foods were fermented: vegetables, meats, fish, milk, fruit, beans, and grains. For most of our existence, we consumed fermented foods every day and received endless health benefits. Since inventing refrigeration and industrial agriculture, we gradually lost the skill of fermentation. This is one of the reasons for the epidemic of abnormal gut flora in modern humans, which leads to many serious consequences. This book will help you to bring these superpower foods back into your life! And they are so easy to make, as Monica shows you in her own wonderful way.
>
> —Dr. Natasha Campbell-McBride

Lacto-Fermentation

Introduction

I wrote the third book in my Cooking Techniques series to focus on one of the pillars of the GAPS diet: lacto-fermented foods and beverages. Because they are fundamental to healing the gut lining, lacto-ferments are required not only in the Intro diet of the GAPS healing protocol but throughout the Full GAPS diet as well. What are lacto-fermented foods and beverages? Why do you need them? When and how do you make them? By the end of this section, you will know the answer to these and many other important questions.

Along the way, we will discuss the wonderfully wide range of starters you can (and should) use for your lacto-ferments. We will explore the nine different methods of fermentation featured in the GAPS diet. And we will delve into the healing powers of the lacto-fermented beverages and tonics that you will need at the beginning of the Intro. From there, we will move on to lacto-fermented vegetables. Before long, you will master all of these lacto-fermented healing foods and possess the knowledge and tools you need to ferment just about anything!

Lacto-ferments are essential to rebuild gut flora and turn the tide on gut dysbiosis. So why wait? Read on to continue your journey to a healed and sealed gut and vibrant digestive health.

Lacto-Fermentation

What Is a Lacto-Ferment?

1

Aren't lacto-ferments made out of milk? Nope. In fact, they are refreshing, healing beverages, tonics, fruits, and vegetables chock-full of what I call "gut good guys," aka beneficial bacteria. You may be familiar with at least two types of lacto-ferments: the crunchy pickles and sauerkraut you find in the refrigerated section of the grocery store. But lacto-ferments are that and so much more.

The *lacto* in "lacto-ferment" has nothing to do with dairy. It stands for lactic acid, which is produced by beneficial bacteria called lactobacilli. In other words, a lacto-ferment is a food or beverage

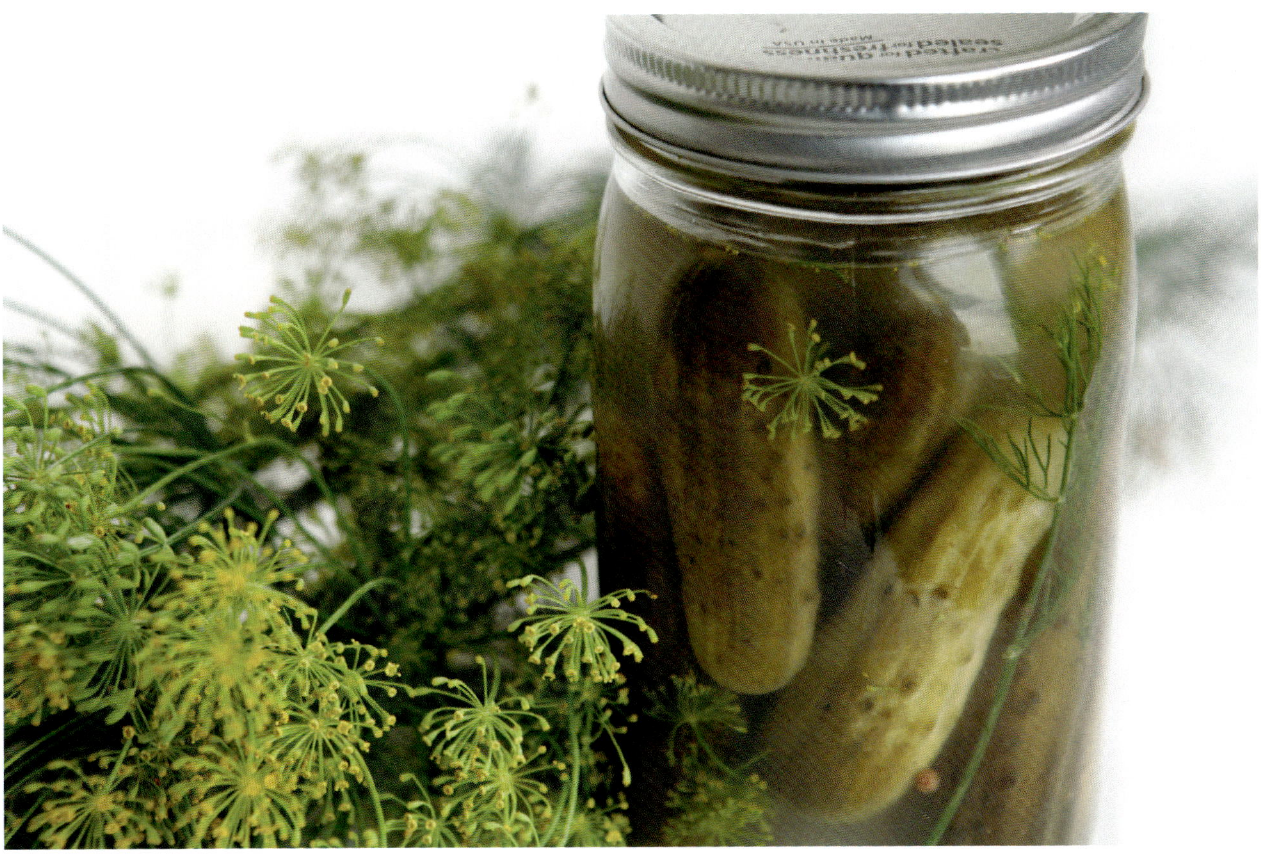

that is fermented by lactic acid-producing bacteria. (For the purposes of the GAPS diet, in this section I will also discuss ferments from lactic acid-producing yeast.)

Some lacto-fermentation recipes do use whey, a protein from dairy, as a starter or inoculant. What if you are dairy intolerant? Have no fear. Even if you experience dairy sensitivities or intolerances, lacto-ferments with whey can still be beneficial for you. And with all of the healing you are doing by following the GAPS diet, you can even begin to overcome your intolerance. (See Section VIII: Culturing Dairy for more specific information.) You can also make many lacto-ferments without using any whey at all.

Don't be fooled: *ferments are powerful foods*. When your body is not used to ferments, consuming too much at a time may provoke a detoxification reaction. If you have never eaten ferments before, or have only eaten them sparingly, start slowly. And by "slowly," I mean as little as a half teaspoon of ferment juice per day, or even a drop of ferment juice diluted in eight ounces of water. It is always important to follow your body's signs. If you experience bloating, flatulence, cramping, diarrhea, constipation, or any other symptoms of imbalance, stay at your current level until the symptoms fade. Only then should you gradually increase the amount. Again, follow your body's lead. If you jump in too quickly, you could develop flu symptoms and wind up in bed for a day or two.

While on the GAPS diet, you will eat and drink many types of lacto-fermented foods and beverages—and a lot of them! Because they add more "gut good guys" to your system, lacto-fermented foods help turn the tide on gut dysbiosis, an imbalance of gut flora caused by too few beneficial bacteria and an overgrowth of bad bacteria. Not only that, but lacto-ferments are true superfoods in many other ways, as you can see from the following list.

The Great and Varied Benefits of Lacto-Fermentation

While the main contribution of lacto-ferments is the addition of beneficial bacteria to your small intestine, the goodness does not stop there. As the following handy-dandy list* shows, lacto-fermentation also:

- Helps "kick on" the digestion process by increasing HCl in the stomach (which aids the digestion of protein)
- Contributes additional enzymes to the digestion process
- Increases vitamin levels, including vitamin C and the B vitamins
- Produces natural antibiotics and anticarcinogenic substances
- Helps the body maintain regular blood pressure and heart rate
- Helps break down fats in the liver
- Helps maintain a healthy level of acidification in the digestive tract
- Promotes growth of healthy bacteria throughout the intestine
- Produces "feel good" substances in the gut
- Boosts immunity

- Decreases levels of pathogenic bacteria (thereby decreasing toxins and cleaning up the gut-brain connection)

Wow! With so many health benefits, why not include these gems in your diet? Especially when they are so inexpensive and easy to make in your own kitchen.

**See sources at the end of this section.*

Lacto-Fermentation

What Is Lacto-Fermentation?

2

Lacto-fermentation is a traditional method of preserving food. It is also one of the oldest—if not *the* oldest. In fact, the earliest record of fermentation dates back as far as 6,000 BC, in a region of the Middle East known as the Fertile Crescent.

But what does it mean to lacto-ferment a food? It means you encourage the growth of healthy bacteria (lactobacilli) that is already present in the food. (Using salt to accomplish this is a centuries-old method of lacto-fermentation that also inhibits the growth of putrefying bacteria.) Or you can *add* healthy bacteria to

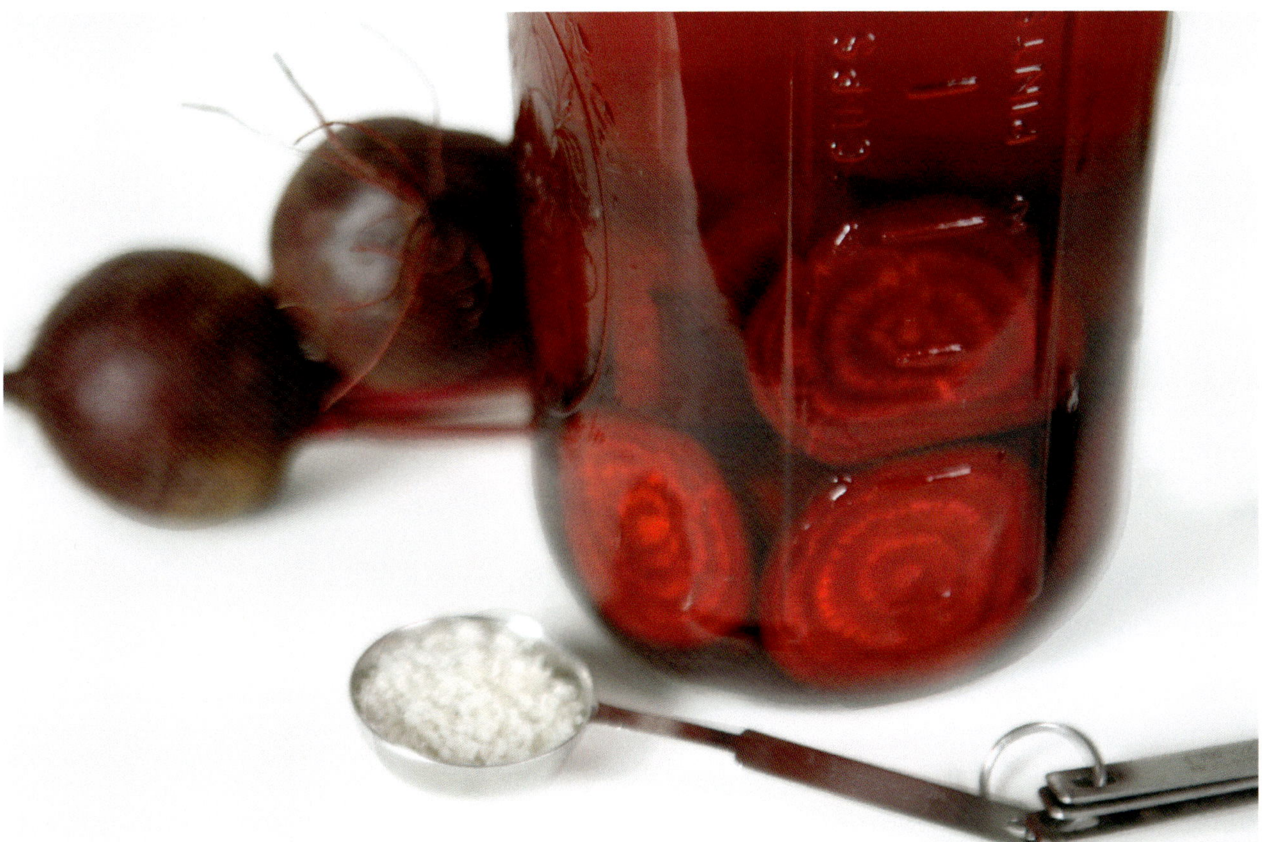

the food or beverage you want to ferment. As the lactobacilli eat the sugars, they give off a natural preservative known as lactic acid.

The process of lacto-fermentation adds enzymes, vitamins, and anticarcinogenic substances to whatever you ferment. Naturally, all of these wonderful things make the food more nutrient rich. Consider lacto-fermentation a value-added process. Not only does it help preserve food, but it also provides you with so many other benefits in the process.

Is Lacto-Fermentation the Same as Canning?

Lacto-fermentation and canning are both methods of preserving food, but that is where the similarities end. Among the major differences between them, the one that matters most is this:

Lacto-fermentation makes food more alive. Canning kills food dead.

What do I mean by "dead"? I mean that the canning process sterilizes food. Sterilization kills enzymes and bacteria—the good kind and the bad—so the food is left nutritionally and enzymatically dead. And without the good bacteria that the sterilization process kills off, the food is also more vulnerable to pathogens. It is not just less healthy. It is also more dangerous.

Canning is a high-heat process that decreases vitamin levels and compromises flavor. What you do gain is shelf life (canned foods are what we call "shelf stable"). In the right conditions, canned foods could sit on your shelf forever, but you lose so much in the process.

Not so with lacto-fermentation. By preserving and adding enzymes, lacto-fermentation makes food more alive. It does everything canning does not: boosts nutrient content, enhances flavor, and improves digestibility. On top of all that, it adds good bacteria and all of the health benefits good bacteria provide.

Hmmm...wouldn't you rather ferment?

There is even more great news about lacto-fermentation. With the addition of a starter, lacto-fermentation can make "dead" foods come "alive" again. Yay!

How does lacto-fermentation bring canned foods back to life? Once you add lactobacilli to canned fruits or vegetables, the bacteria get to work. They begin to eat the sugars. The lactobacilli predigest the cellulose for you. They create all of the wonderful vitamins and nutrients for which lacto-fermented foods are so well known. And once you lacto-ferment a canned food, you get many of the other health benefits we discussed in the previous chapter. (However, it is important to note that the nutrient content in canned food will still be compromised even after you lacto-ferment it. But the addition of live bacteria makes it that much better for you to eat and easier to digest.)

How does it work? In a real-world example, say you would like to make your own condiments, such as lacto-fermented ketchup. Instead of using the canned (dead) tomato paste from the recipe, you lacto-ferment it first. Now it is no longer "dead." The process of fermenting the tomato paste results in an enzyme-rich ketchup that is full of lactobacilli!

Lacto-Fermentation vs. Canning

	Lacto-Fermentation	Canning
Contains live bacteria	√	
Predigests food	√	
Predigests sugar	√	
Predigests fiber/cellulose	√	
Increases vitamin and nutrient content	√	
Produces anti-cancer substances	√	
Produces natural antibiotic substances	√	
Helps normalize blood pressure	√	
Helps normalize blood sugar	√	
Boosts immune system function	√	
Enhances flavor	√	
Can be stored at room temperature		√
Uses heat		√
Kills enzymes		√
Sterilizes		√
Decreases vitamin and nutrient content		√

See Sources at the end of this section.

Is Lacto-Fermentation the Same as Pickling?

We just covered the pros and cons of canning vs. lacto-fermentation. But there is yet another method of preserving food: pickling. Like canning, pickling is inferior to lacto-fermentation because it does not yield lactobacilli. Only lacto-fermentation can do that. This is important to keep in mind because lactobacilli are not only good for you but also required for the GAPS diet.

Lacto-fermentation is an anaerobic process that involves the addition of brine (salt and water) to foster a beneficial environment that encourages the growth of lactobacilli. Lacto-fermentation can also involve the addition of lactobacilli in the form of a starter or inoculant. As the lactobacilli grow, they give off lactic acid, which preserves the food.

Pickling, on the other hand, involves the use of either brine or vinegar (usually vinegar and sugar). Foods pickled in vinegar do not grow good bacteria. In fact, commercially available pickled foods are often pasteurized (that is, sterilized) before they hit the shelf at the supermarket. That means pickled foods can be just as enzymatically and nutritionally "dead" as canned foods.

We also need to consider sugar in pickling vs. lacto-fermenting. In lacto-fermented foods, the lactobacilli eat the sugars. But in pickled foods, sugar can be added as part of the recipe.

All of this makes it clear that pickled foods do not have the same healthful benefits as lacto-fermented foods—and that is why they are not part of the GAPS diet. The focus here is strictly on lacto-fermentation. Even when it comes to "pickles," we are really talking about *lacto-fermented* cucumbers!

Lacto-Fermentation

Why Make Your Own Lacto-Ferments?

3

I am often asked if store-bought ferments are okay on the GAPS diet. For reasons that will soon become clear, my answer is that you should stay away from store-bought ferments whenever you can. However, if you are in a pinch (for example, while traveling) and cannot make your own, eating store-bought ferments is better than not eating ferments at all. Store-bought ferments are also a handy choice when you are just starting out on your journey to good gut health and have not yet learned how to make your own. (But this section will remedy that!)

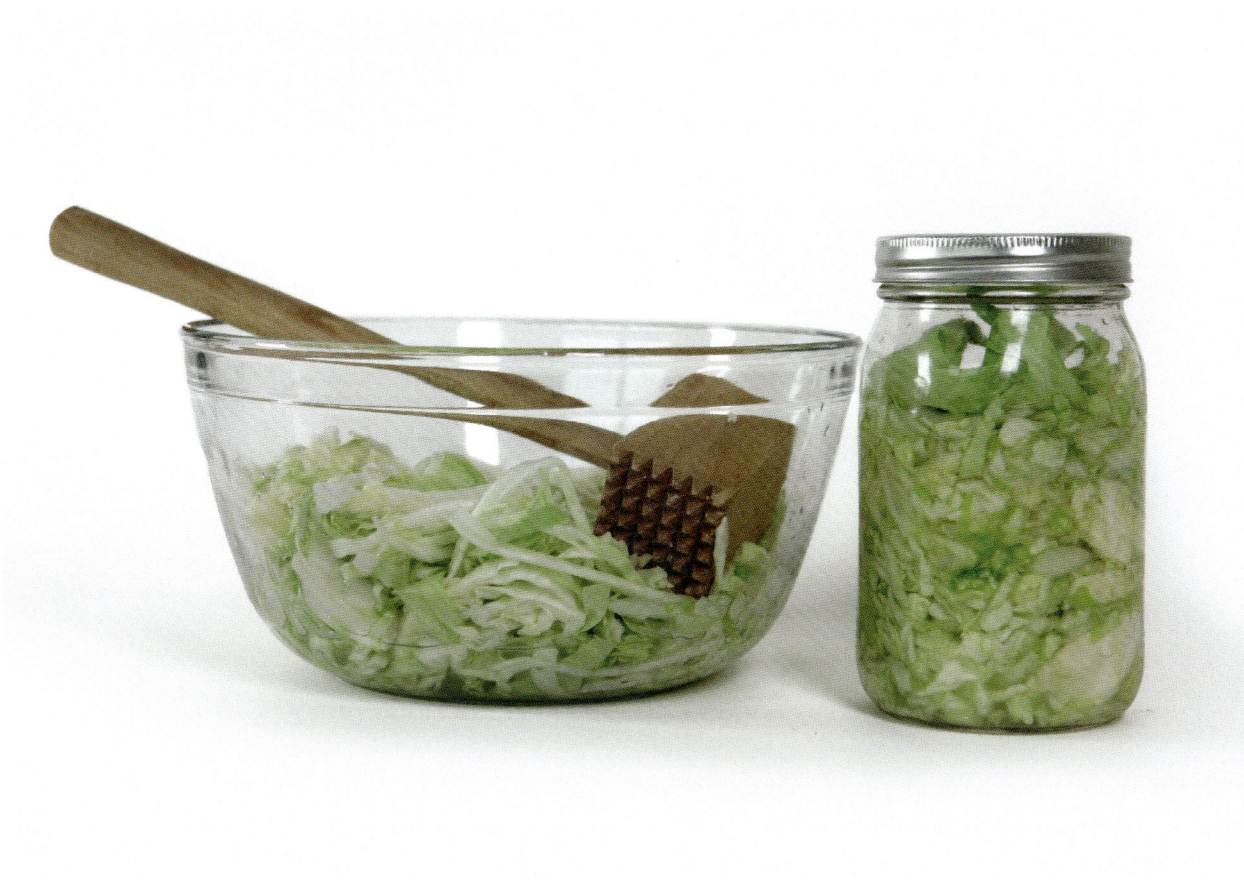

Eventually, you will want to be the master of your own ferments. Store-bought ferments are simply not as good for you, especially if you have a permeable or leaky gut. Read on to learn why.

Say No to Store-Bought Ferments

Many ferments in the grocery store have been lightly pasteurized to give them a longer shelf life. Unfortunately, after pasteurization takes place you cannot tell how "live" with lactobacilli the ferments are. Why gamble with your health when you can make your own robust and varied ferments instead?

Additionally, most store-bought ferments are made from conventionally grown rather than organic vegetables. This is highly problematic. If you are on the GAPS diet, you have a leaky gut. If you have a leaky gut, toxins are already flooding your brain and liver. You definitely cannot afford any additional toxins in your diet! Yet, if you purchase store-bought ferments that contain conventionally grown ingredients, that is exactly what you will get. If, on the other hand, you make your own ferments, you can avoid conventional produce altogether. No conventional produce means no toxic pesticide residues to hamper the process of lacto-fermentation.

Which leads us to an even more problematic issue. When we talk about conventional ingredients, we are talking about the state of our food supply at large. GMOs are cropping up everywhere. Many GMO products are not yet labeled, which makes it next to impossible to avoid them. Harmful chemical pesticides, herbicides, and fungicides abound. In fact, conventional farmers sprayed more than five million pounds of these dangerous substances on their fields in 2006. In the following year, the estimate was more than *one billion pounds* (Environmental Protection Agency, "Pesticides Industry Sales and Usage: 2006 and 2007 Market Estimates," February 2011). No matter how much you scrub or rinse your fruits and vegetables, these toxins will inevitably wind up in your ferments. Therefore, if your gut needs healing, you will do well to make your own ferments with organic fruits and vegetables. And you have choices! You can buy certified organic produce, grow it yourself, or get it from a farmer you trust.

When it comes to produce, there are some fruits and vegetables that are even more important to buy organic than others. To learn the difference, check out the annual Dirty Dozen and Clean Fifteen reports put out by the Environmental Working Group (EWG). The Dirty Dozen is a list of twelve conventionally grown fruits and vegetables that contain the *most* toxic load of pesticide residue, while the Clean Fifteen is a list of fifteen conventionally grown fruits and vegetables that are *least* likely to contain pesticide residues.

What does this mean for you? Simply put, it is worthwhile to spend your organic dollars on the Dirty Dozen list. But when you must buy conventionally grown produce, stick with the safer options from the Clean Fifteen list.

Benefits of Making Your Own Lacto-Ferments

In addition to all of the great reasons for avoiding store-bought ferments that I discuss above, here are even more ways you benefit by making your lacto-ferments:

- You ensure that only high-quality, organic ingredients are in your lacto-ferments.
- You control how long you want the fermentation process to take—and therefore how potent your ferments will be.
- You get to use many different types of starters to guarantee a good variety of lactobacilli (more on starters in the next chapter).
- You can look forward to eating your creations because they will taste great!

Lacto-Fermentation

All About Starters

4

What is a starter? Before we answer that question, perhaps we should go back to the beginning. Before starters. As previously mentioned, lacto-fermentation has been around for a long time, since 6,000 BC or so. Back then, the original recipe for lacto-fermentation involved salt, and to this day salt continues to be all you really need to lacto-ferment a food or beverage. Salt not only sets up the conditions that allow lactobacilli to grow, but it also prevents the growth of putrefying bacteria. But if salt is all we need, why add a starter at all?

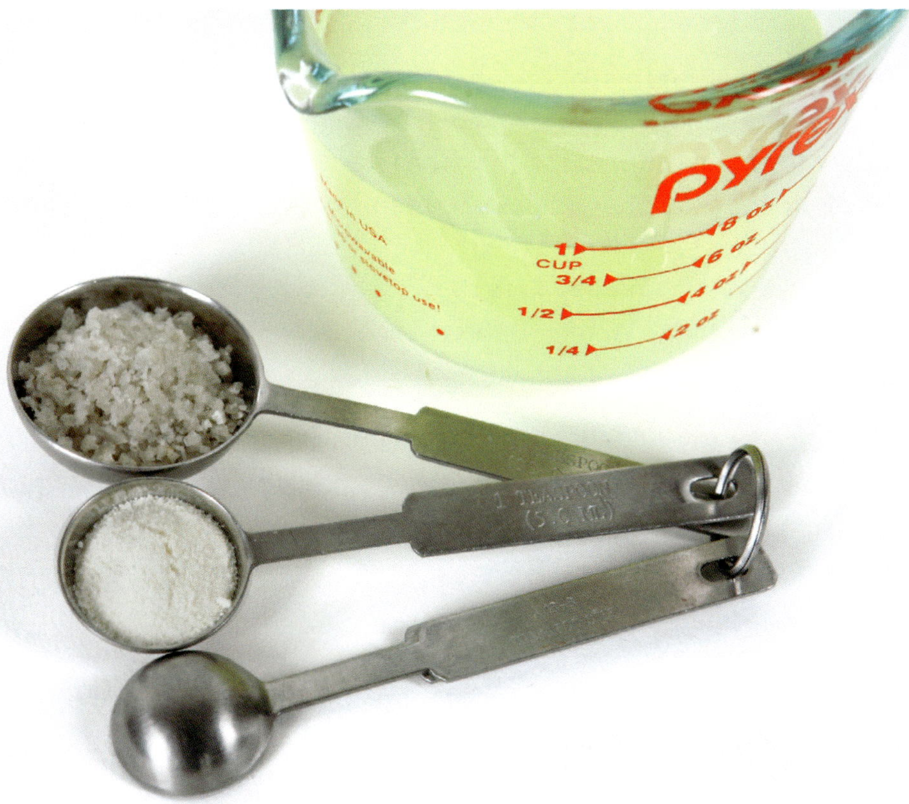

Think of starters as an insurance policy that lacto-fermentation will happen, and happen quickly. You can also lacto-ferment a food by adding a starter in addition to salt. Or, if you use enough of it, in place of salt. Starters are also known as "inoculants" or "fermentation agents." You inoculate whatever you are lacto-fermenting with lactobacilli. Then the starter does just what you think it does: it "starts" or "kick-starts" the lacto-fermentation process. As you explore the various types of starters, keep in mind that you can also lacto-ferment the same way we have been doing it for centuries, with the use of salt alone.

However, starters—especially when you use a variety of them—are very important in the GAPS healing protocol. Read on to learn what they are, what makes them so crucial, and where and how to obtain them.

Types of Starters for Lacto-Fermentation

Below is a list of starters you can use in lacto-fermentation. You can find the starter packets mentioned below at grocery stores or online. And in Section VIII: Culturing Dairy you will find recipes for making your own whey three different ways! (This is important as you should never buy powdered whey.)

- Whey strained from yogurt
- Whey strained from kefir
- Whey from separating raw milk*
- Whey from cheese-making (if you make your own cheese)
- Ferment juice (from a previous ferment)
- Starter packet for making yogurt
- Starter packet for making kefir
- Starter packet for making cultured vegetables
- Probiotic capsule of lactobacilli

*If you have access to raw milk, this makes a great starter. **But you must not substitute pasteurized milk for raw milk to make whey under *any* circumstances.** You can end up very sick.

The Importance of Using Different Starters

I highly recommended using multiple starters throughout the GAPS healing protocol, both in the Intro and in the Full GAPS diet. Why? Because the more starters you use for your ferments, the more likely you will achieve a broader profile of multispecies, flourishing gut flora (lactobacilli). And, presumably, the faster you will heal.

As you can see, starters come in many forms. Each time you make a different recipe, try changing up the starter you use.

Lacto-Fermentation

Introducing Lacto-Fermented Beverages and Vegetables

5

In the GAPS healing protocol, you generally introduce lacto-ferments right from the start of the Intro diet, in Stage 1. However, you do not start with lacto-fermented foods at this point—those will come later. In the Intro you start with the "juice" of ferments (for example, the brine from sauerkraut or lacto-fermented pickles).

Within a short amount of time of beginning the Intro, you will work your way up to needing a quarter to a half cup of ferment juice *per meal*. That is a lot of ferment juice! If you were to get

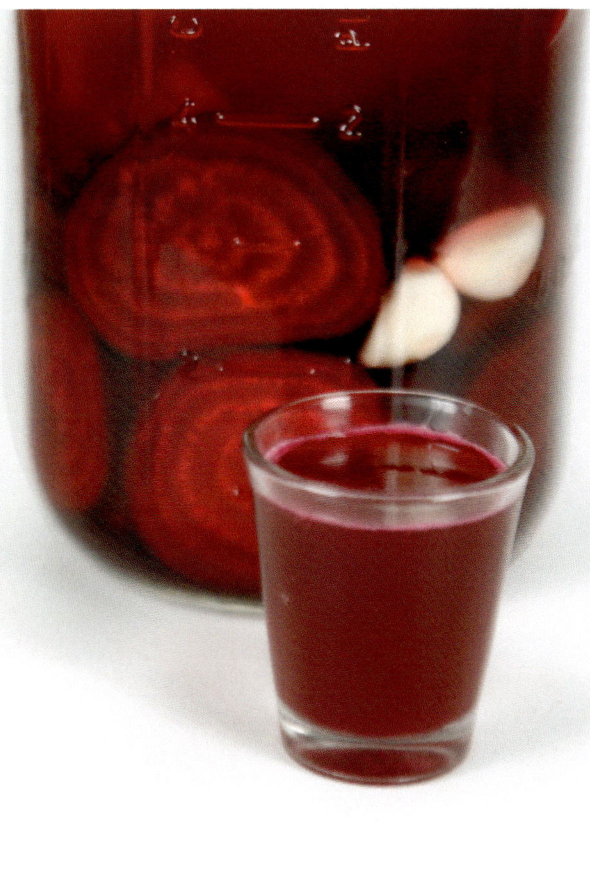

your ferment juice from kraut and pickles alone, you would have to prepare a lot of kraut and pickles. (And you cannot even eat them yet!) To prevent this, I suggest a work-around.

Sauerkraut and pickles are both examples of fermented vegetables that provide ferment juice (even though pickles are really fermented cucumbers, which are technically a fruit.) But a full quart of kraut will only yield a few ounces of the ferment juice you need during the Intro. So instead of preparing fermented vegetables at all, I suggest you start off by making lacto-fermented *beverages* (including tonics) instead. Voila! This is a far easier way to ensure you have as much ferment juice as you need.

Why Start with Ferment Juice?

You may be wondering why you need to start with ferment juice at all. Why not simply begin with fermented fruits and vegetables? The answer is in your gut lining, which can be injured by consuming fermented fruits and vegetables too early on in the GAPS healing protocol. (Think of sandpaper on an open wound.) The Intro diet is meant to be a healing and rebuilding diet. As such, foods that could be hard on your digestive system are not included. In order to give your gut the best possible chance of healing and rebuilding, you begin with the most easily digested foods, including easily digestible ferment juice.

As you progress through the six stages of the Intro diet, your system will become stronger. You will gradually be able to digest more challenging foods: cabbage in the case of sauerkraut, cucumbers in the case of pickles, to name just two. But not in the beginning. As you start the Intro, put those more challenging foods aside. You will get the ferments into your diet in the amounts you need with ferment juice alone. To this end, you will find recipes for the fermented beverages (Fruit or Vegetable Kvass) and tonics (Beet Kvass) you need in chapter 9.

Lacto-Ferments at a Glance

Type of Lacto-Ferment	Ingredients	Examples	Best Time to Eat	Benefits & Challenges
Beverages	Vegetables, fruits, or combination **Choose one:** 1) Salt 2) Salt and starter 3) Starter alone	Vegetable and/or Fruit kvass*	**Best:** Stages 1 and 2 of Intro **Good:** Intro and Full GAPS diet	**Benefits:** Liquid No fiber to digest No early injury to GI tract
Tonics	Beets **Choose one:** 1) Salt 2) Salt and starter	Beet kvass*	**Best:** Stages 1 and 2 of Intro **Good:** Intro and Full GAPS diet	**Benefits:** Liquid No fiber to digest No early injury to GI tract Tonics are especially healing to the body
Vegetables	Vegetables **Choose one:** 1) Salt 2) Salt and starter	Sauerkraut* Kimchi Lacto-fermented pickles and beets (aka "pickled" beets) Gingered carrots	**Best:** Start at Stage 3 of Intro **Continue:** Stages 4–6 and Full GAPS diet	**Challenges:** Fiber can be injurious early on in the Intro (waiting until Stage 3 is best)
Fruits	Fruit **Choose one:** 1) Salt 2) Salt and starter	Lacto-fermented berries Chutneys Apple/pear sauce or butter	**Best:** Start at Stage 5 of Intro **Continue:** Stage 6 and Full GAPS diet	**Challenges:** Fiber and possible sugar content (if it does not ferment fully)

**See Chapter 9: The Recipes.*

Lacto-Fermentation

Important Facts to Remember

6

Keep the following in mind as you make your ferments for the GAPS diet, and you will soon become an expert!

Add liquid to cover. Always be sure to add enough liquid (brine) to cover your ingredients. If the vegetables or fruits are not sufficiently covered with liquid, mold can develop. Exceptions include lacto-fermented ketchup, mustard, apple butter, and other ferments made from purees. These do not use water, so you do not need to keep them covered.

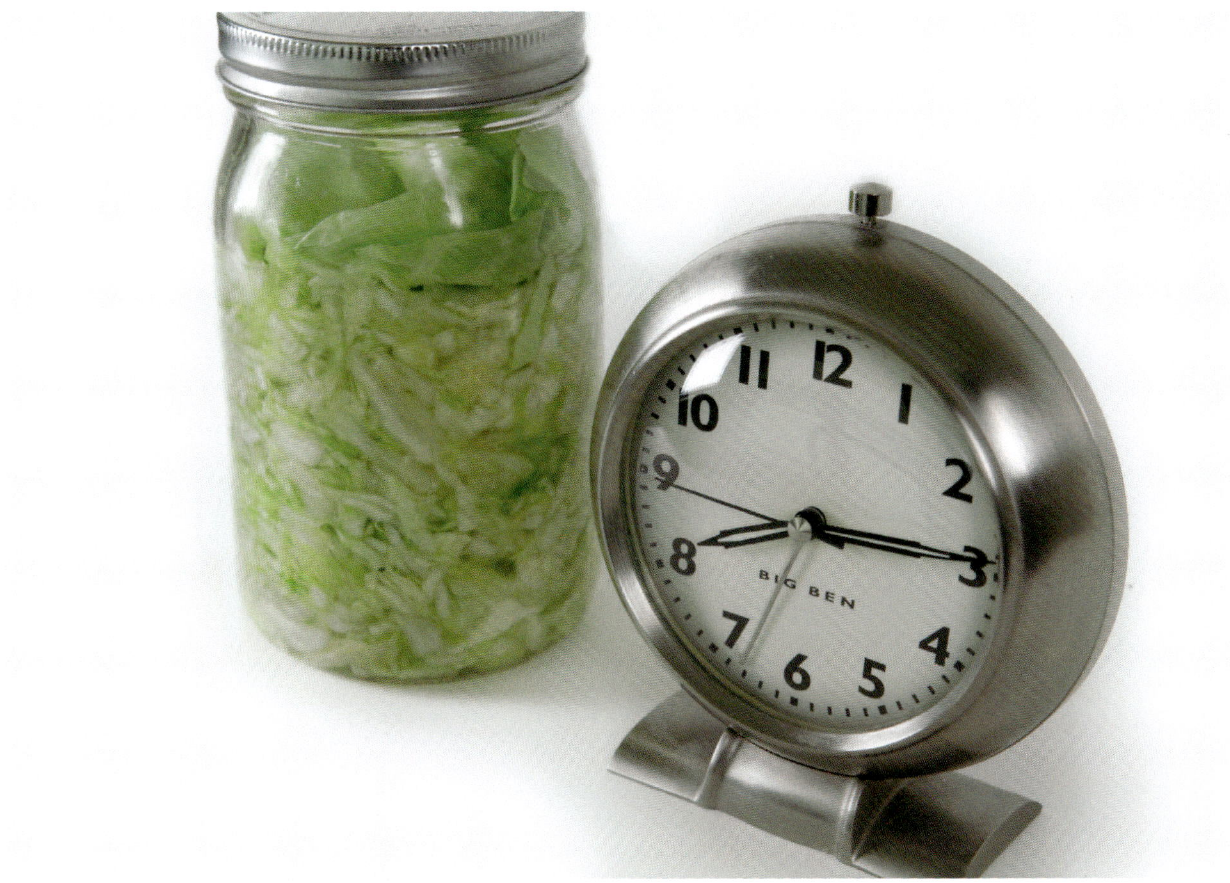

Do not open jar. Fermentation is an anaerobic process. Too much oxygen will ruin the vegetables or fruit, resulting in putrefaction rather than lacto-fermentation. To avoid this, do not open the jar until the process is over.

Leave enough space. Be sure to leave about two inches of space between the top of the vegetables and the top of the jar. If you are using a wide-mouth, 1-quart or 2-quart jar, this space often starts at the "shoulder," where the jar curves. Leaving two inches allows for the natural expansion of the vegetables as the lactobacilli digest the sugars and release lactic acid. It also prevents leaks.

Ferment at room temperature. Allow fermentation to happen at room temperature (68–72°F). The temperature of the room directly impacts how quickly or slowly your food ferments. The cooler the room, the longer it takes. The hotter the room, the faster.

Sugar content and fermentation time. The speed of fermentation also depends on the sugar content of the food. The higher the sugar content of your vegetables or fruit, the faster the fermentation process. Likewise, the lower the sugar content, the slower the process. For example, fruit ferments very quickly, while cabbage, which is low in sugar, takes the longest to ferment.

Sugar content and shelf life. Sugar content also impacts shelf life (usually the shelf in your refrigerator). The higher the sugar content, the shorter the shelf life. The lower the sugar content, the longer the shelf life. Again, fermented fruit will have a shorter shelf life than fermented cabbage (aka sauerkraut).

Storage temperature. When your ferments are done, place them in cold storage (40°F or so). A root cellar, a small refrigerator kept on warm, or the top shelf of your refrigerator (usually the warmest spot) should all work.

Storage time. Lacto-fermented vegetables and low-sugar fruits such as cucumbers and tomatoes keep several months in cold storage. Lacto-fermented fruits and preserves should be eaten within two months.

Bubbles. Some lacto-fermented fruits and vegetables may get bubbly. This is natural.

Foam. Harmless white spots or foam may appear on the top of your pickling liquid. Simply remove with a spoon.

For more information, see Chapter 10: Frequently Asked Questions.

Lacto-Fermentation

The Techniques

7

The GAPS diet encourages you to try as many different methods of fermentation as possible. The more methods you use, the greater variety of lactobacilli (gut good guys) you will introduce to your digestive system. So mix it up! As Dr. Natasha Campbell-McBride says, "The more the merrier. And healthier, too!"

The nine different methods of lacto-fermentation discussed below are all variations on a theme: creating an anaerobic environment that encourages the growth of lactobacilli. Some of these methods are specific to the GAPS diet, especially in terms of salt quantity, starter type, and fermentation time.

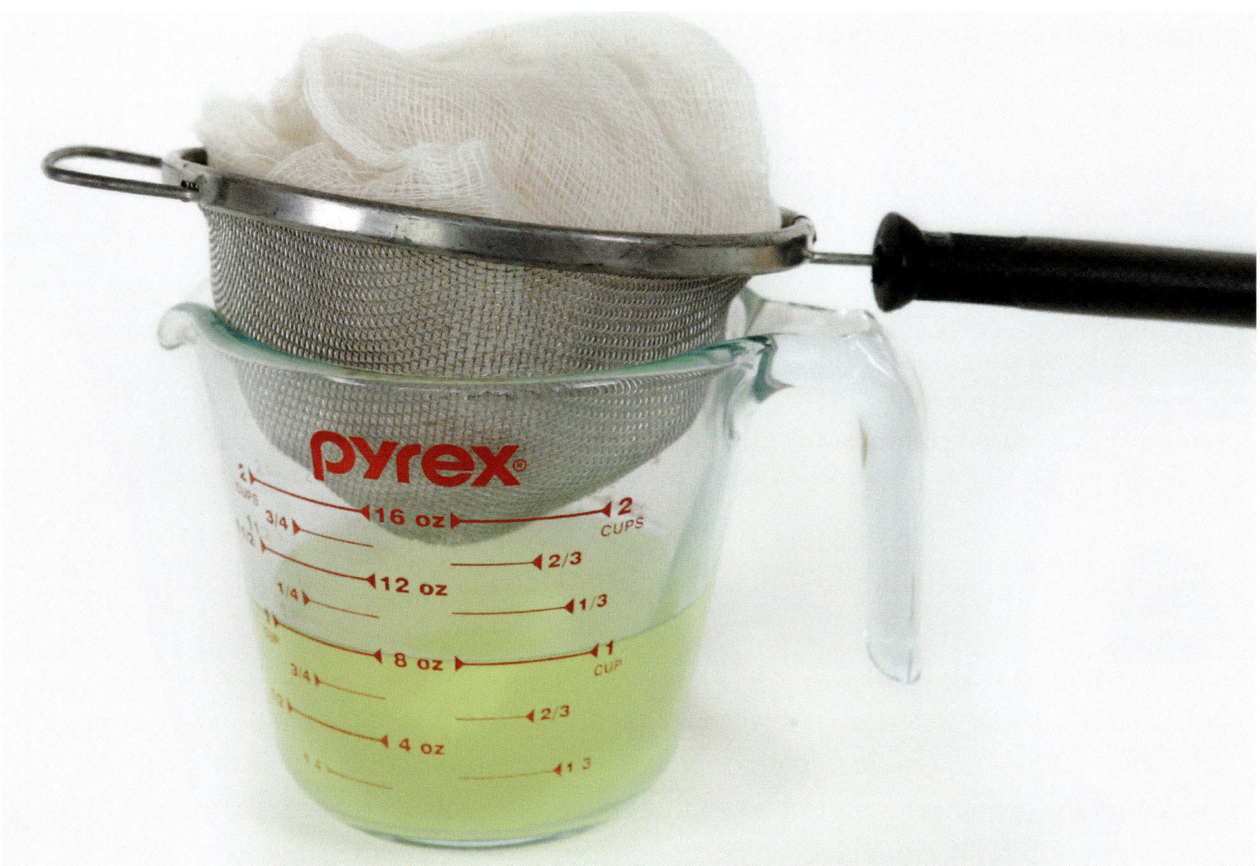

As previously noted, fermenting with salt alone is the original, centuries-old recipe. Salt plays a very important role in setting up conditions for lactobacilli to grow. However, in some of the methods below, salt is not used at all. Instead, you over-inoculate the ferment by using much more starter than you would if you were using salt alone. I call this "inoculating high," and it is outlined in methods 6 and 7 below.

A note on fermentation time: If you ferment more than a quart jar at a time, you will need to extend the fermentation time. The more food you ferment, the longer it will take. (This principle does not apply to beverages.) For example, if you ferment a ½-gallon to 1-gallon jar of vegetables, you will need to extend your fermentation time to 1–2 weeks.

Variety Is the Spice of Life! 9 Methods of Lacto-Fermentation Encouraged by the GAPS Diet

Who needs recipes when you have templates? The following list will help you ferment just about any ingredient you like in a variety of ways. You cannot get it wrong if you follow these easy guidelines, so try them all!

Also note that for culinary purposes the term "vegetables" includes tomatoes, cucumbers, zucchini, and other low-sugar fruits.

You will find more information on making your own whey from kefir, yogurt, and raw milk (as called for in #3, #6, and #7) in Section VIII: Culturing Dairy. Always use filtered watered whenever water is called for. And remember, never use powdered whey.

#1. Salt Alone (aka "Salt Solo") Fermentation

Ingredients: Vegetables and salt alone. This method usually applies only to sauerkraut or ferments made with cabbage (the cabbage itself supplies the water needed to cover).

Basic recipe: For every quart of vegetables, add 1–2 tablespoons sea salt. Pack into a quart jar up to the shoulder, leaving plenty of room for expansion as the cabbage ferments. Ferment 5–7 days at room temperature, or until the lid is taut. (If you prefer a milder sauerkraut, you may leave it for 2 weeks or more, as long as you have enough room in the jar for expansion.)

#2. Fermentation with Brine

Ingredients: Vegetables and brine (salt and water) to cover.

Basic recipe: For every quart of vegetables, add 1–2 tablespoons sea salt. Pack into a quart jar up to the shoulder. Cover with water, leaving about 2 inches of room for expansion. Ferment 5–7 days at room temperature, or until the lid is taut.

#3. Fermentation with Brine and Whey

Ingredients: Vegetables, brine (salt and water), and whey (from yogurt or kefir, or from separating raw—never pasteurized—milk).

Basic recipe: For every quart of vegetables, add 1–2 teaspoons salt (or to taste). Fill a quart jar halfway with the vegetables. Add ½ cup whey. Cover with water, leaving about 2 inches of space between the vegetables and the lid. Ferment for 1 week at room temperature, or until the lid is taut.

#4. Fermentation with Yogurt or Kefir Starter

Ingredients: Vegetables, brine (salt and water), and a yogurt starter or kefir starter (from a starter packet).

Basic recipe: For every quart of vegetables, dissolve 1 packet of yogurt or kefir starter in 2 cups of water. Stir. Salt vegetables to taste (1–2 teaspoons) and place them in a quart jar to the shoulder. Cover with water-starter mixture, leaving about 2 inches of space between vegetables and lid. Ferment for 1 week at room temperature, or until the lid is taut.

#5. Fermentation with Vegetable Starter

Ingredients: Vegetables, brine (salt and water), and vegetable starter (from a starter packet).

Basic recipe: For every quart of vegetables, dissolve 1 packet of vegetable starter in 2 cups of water. Stir. Salt vegetables to taste (1–2 teaspoons) and place them in a quart jar to the shoulder. Cover with water-starter mixture, leaving about 2 inches of space between vegetables and lid. Ferment for 1 week at room temperature, or until the lid is taut.

#6. Fermentation with Whey Alone

Ingredients: Beverage or tonic and whey (from yogurt or kefir, or from separating raw—never pasteurized—milk).

Basic recipe: Pour ½ cup whey into a quart jar. Fill jar to shoulder with beverage or tonic. Cover tightly with lid. Ferment for 1 week at room temperature, or until the lid is taut. (For a 2-quart jar, you may easily double the basic recipe.)

#7. Fermentation with Whey and Water

Ingredients: Vegetables, water, and whey (from yogurt or kefir, or from separating raw—never pasteurized—milk).

Basic recipe: Pour ½ cup whey into a quart jar. Fill jar to shoulder with vegetables. Cover with water, leaving about 2 inches of space between vegetables and lid. Ferment for 1 week at room temperature, or until the lid is taut.

#8. Fermentation Using Previous Batch

Ingredients: Vegetables, brine (from a previous batch of fermented vegetables), beverage or tonic, and water.

Basic recipe: For every quart of vegetables, use ¼ cup of brine from a previous batch. Fill a quart jar to the shoulder with vegetables. Cover with additional water. Ferment for 1 week at room temperature, or until the lid is taut.

#9. Fermentation Using a Probiotic

Ingredients: Vegetables, brine, and a probiotic (lactobacilli) capsule.

Basic recipe: For every quart of vegetables, stir 1 one probiotic capsule in 2 cups of water to dissolve. Salt vegetables to taste (1–2 teaspoons) and place in a quart jar. Cover vegetables with water-probiotic mixture. Ferment for 1 week at room temperature, or until the lid is taut.

Lacto-Fermentation

Jars, Bowls, and Crocks!

8

You can use many different vessels for lacto-fermentation. The original method involved ceramic crocks or jars, which would be filled with vegetables, sprinkled with salt, and covered. For our purposes, we will mostly use wide-mouthed glass jars with two-piece lids—especially when making lacto-fermented beverages or tonics, for sure. However, you may also use bowls or crocks specifically designed for lacto-fermentation. The following section explains more about when and why to use a jar, bowl, or crock for fermenting.

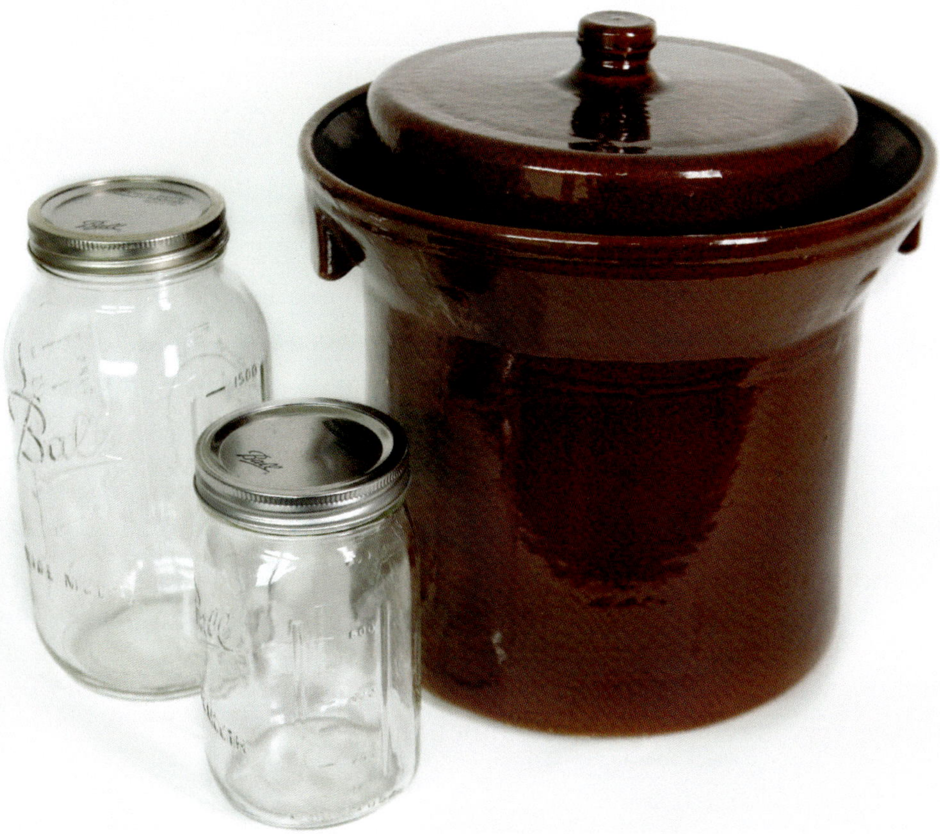

Jar Fermentation

The fermentation process I use is called the "jar method." As you may have guessed, it uses jars! This method of fermentation is relatively quick because you ferment a small amount at a time (a quart or half-gallon). Jars are efficient: they take up a small amount of space, and you can store your ferment in the same vessel you make it in. Purchasing wide-mouth canning jars with two-piece lids in various sizes is the least expensive way to ferment in jars.

The recipes in chapter 9 call for one-quart and two-quart (½-gallon) jars. In general, the jar method for lacto-fermentation takes anywhere from two days to two weeks, depending on the ingredient and the temperature. (Remember, the warmer the room, the faster the ferment.)

Recent years have also seen the rise of "fermentation locks" or "airlocks." These were traditionally used for making beer or wine but have since been adapted for vegetable ferments. Fermentation locks are another version of jar fermentation, but the airlock system draws the oxygen out of the jar. This creates a truly anaerobic environment for your ferments and speeds up the fermentation process.

Bowl or Crock Fermentation

You also have the option of using a fermentation crock or a bowl with a plate on top (the plate should be just one centimeter smaller than the bowl). If you decide on a crock, make sure to get one with a water seal. Water seal crocks come in 1-gallon, 5-liter, 10-liter, 15-liter, and up to 40-liter (10-gallon) sizes.

Avoid "open crocks" as they can yield less predictable results and are also more prone to mold and yeast. We do not want mold and yeast to grow. We want lactobacilli to grow. As mentioned, lactobacilli are anaerobic. They do not like oxygen, which is why open crocks are not recommended for lacto-fermentation in the GAPS diet.

Crocks were widely used prior to jars and lids, making them one of the oldest methods of fermentation. They are most useful for fermenting a large amount of vegetables at a time. But keep in mind: the larger the volume, the longer the fermentation time. Depending on the volume, it can take up to 6 months or more to lacto-ferment your vegetables.

Whichever method you use—jar, crock, or bowl—be sure to keep whatever you are fermenting submerged under an adequate amount of brine!

Jar vs. Crock Fermentation

	Jar	Crock
Volume	Low volume: ½ pint to 1 gallon	High volume: 5 gallons or more
Time	2–14 days on average	6 months or more
Space	Need small amount of space (depending on size)	Need enough space to fit a large crock
Odor	No odor (jar remains closed)	Some odor (crock is not truly sealed)
Weight	Relatively light	Heavy (crock contains large volume of vegetables and water)
Storage	Ferment already stored in jar	Must transfer fermented vegetables to jars for storage; cannot store in crock

Recommended Fermentation Crocks for High Volume Fermentation

- Harsch Gartopf Fermenting Crock
- Nik Schmitt Fermenting Crock
- Bristol Fermenting Crock

Handy Kitchen Utensils for Lacto-Fermentation

- Wide-mouth mason jars in 1-pint, 1-quart, and 2-quart (½-gallon) sizes, or a fermentation crock (if using a crock, you will also need mason jars for storage)
- Canning lids to fit jars (2-piece lids are best)
- Measuring spoons (especially a tablespoon)
- 2-cup liquid measure, glass preferred
- Fine mesh strainer to fit in 2-cup liquid measure
- Cheesecloth, lint-free tea towels, or nut bags
- Large, stainless steel bowl
- Large wooden or bamboo cutting board
- Sharp chef's knife
- Meat pounder (wooden or metal)
- Canning funnel

You may also want:

- Airlock system and lid
- Fermentation weights, pie weights, or smaller jars (to keep vegetables submerged)
- Sharpie (for labeling and marking dates on jars)

Lacto-Fermentation

9 The Recipes

Woo-hoo! Congratulations! You have now learned all you need to know about lacto-fermentation: what it is, how it works, what different starters to use, and which ferments to start with. Now it is time for some recipes. While these will stand you in good stead for your journey through the Intro and the Full GAPS diet (and beyond), I hope you will use your new knowledge to make many other lacto-fermented beverages, vegetables, and fruits. Remember, fermented foods and beverages are part of a healthy diet that will help ensure a strong immune system over your lifetime.

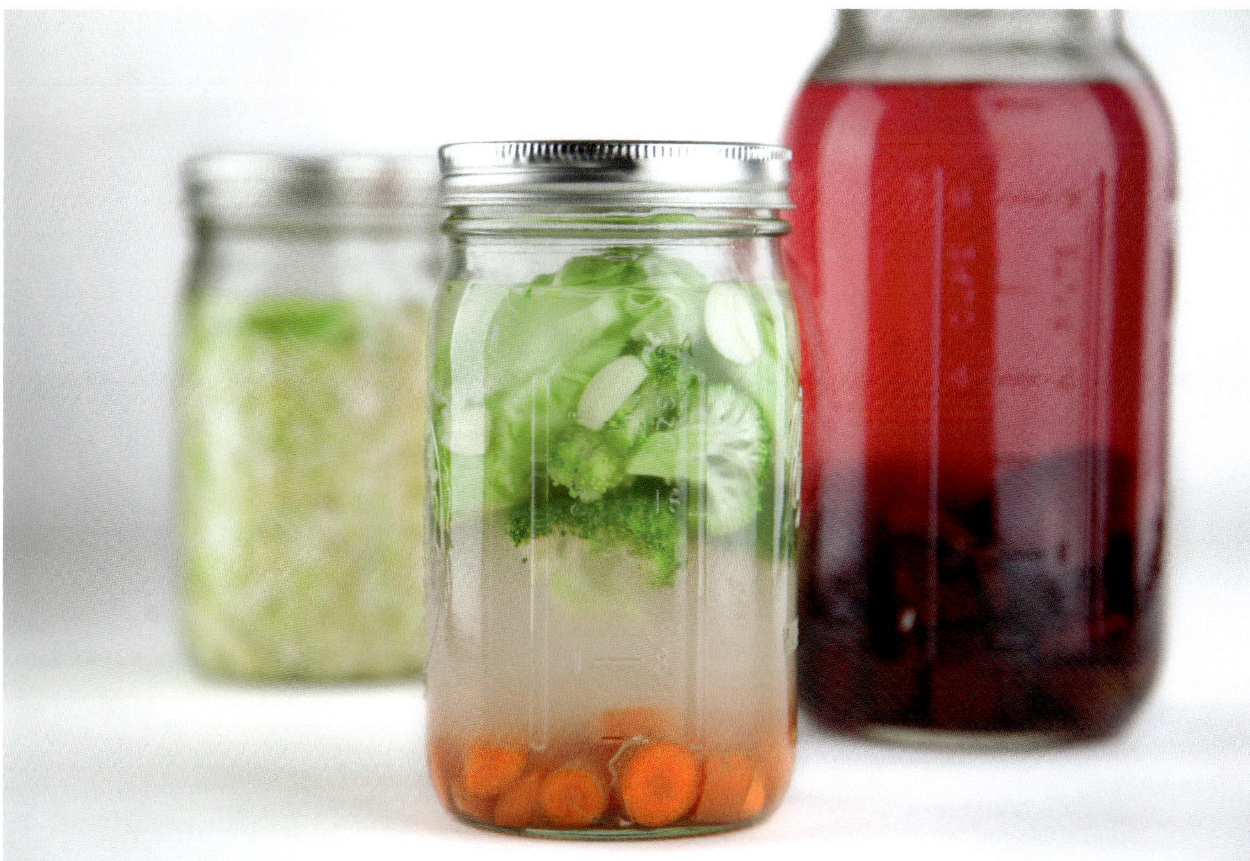

Before you begin any of these recipes, review the following list to ensure success. Happy fermenting!

5 Things You Need to Successfully Ferment a Food

1. *Time:* Two to three days to two weeks, or even longer if you use a crock.
2. *Temperature:* Ferment at room temperature (68–72°F).
3. *Sea salt:* Use a high-quality, fine sea salt for your lacto-ferments and for the GAPS diet in general (Celtic Sea Salt is a good choice). As Dr. Natasha Campbell-McBride makes clear, most people on GAPS have mineral deficiencies, so using sea salt with no fillers or anti-caking agents is essential. To learn more, visit SeleneRiverPress.com and check out "Eat Your Salt" by Stephanie Selene Anderson.
4. *Starter:* Also known as an inoculant or fermenting agent, starters include whey from homemade yogurt, kefir, or raw (never pasteurized) milk. Because whey proteins are easily denatured, powdered whey is not recommended. You may also use a kefir or yogurt starter packet, a vegetable starter packet, brine from a previous batch, or a probiotic. Remember, starters are optional but highly recommended.
5. *Jar, bowl, or crock:* You will need one of the following vessels: a wide-mouth glass jar with a two-piece lid; a bowl with a plate just one centimeter smaller; or a crock.

Some Notes on Whey

As mentioned above, whey may be used as a starter or inoculant for your lacto-ferments. Section VIII: Culturing Dairy features recipes on how to make whey three ways: from yogurt, kefir, or raw milk (never pasteurized). Please note: Whey should be clear, without any milk solids in it. If you have milk solids in your whey, simply strain again.

Also keep in mind that kefir produces a stronger die-off reaction than yogurt. For your lacto-ferments, you may wish to start with whey from yogurt and work your way to using whey from kefir. If possible, using homemade kefir is best.

Lacto-Fermented Beverages and Tonics for the Intro Diet

The following recipes for lacto-fermented beverages and tonics are especially useful for the Intro part of the GAPS diet, though you may of course use them throughout the GAPS healing protocol and even after you transition off the diet. As I stated previously, you start with the most easily digested foods during the stages of the Intro diet, and then you gradually work up to foods that are more challenging to digest.

During the Intro you will be adding the juice of ferments (aka fermented beverages or tonics) to every cup of meat stock, soup, or stew that you drink or eat. Eventually you will work your way up to about a quarter cup per meal—almost a cup a day, or a quart of ferment juice every four days or so. That is why I recommend preparing lacto-fermented beverages and tonics rather than try to achieve the same goal with a jar of sauerkraut, especially since you cannot even eat the kraut itself until Stage 3 (which may take a few months).

For all of your ferments, let me emphasize how important it is to use high-quality ingredients. Remember, you are making *healing foods*, so take care to use organic vegetables and fruits whenever possible. You do not want your body to expend energy countering toxins from conventionally grown produce.

> This also bears repeating: it is essential to use good water for your ferments! What is "good" water? Sadly, it does not pour out of your tap. Tap water contains added chemicals that kill the very bacteria you are trying to grow. So stay away from the tap and use spring or filtered water instead.

Fruit or Vegetable Kvass

You can make kvass (which simply means "fermented drink") a variety of ways: from a vegetable or a combination of vegetables; from fruits and berries; or from any combination of the two. Dr. Natasha also suggests (and I agree) that it is nice to add garlic or ginger. Be creative with your combinations until you find just the flavor profile you love!

Children tend to love fruit kvass, so this is a good place to start if you have kids. When making fruit kvass, keep in mind that low-sugar berries (blueberries, blackberries, and raspberries) work best. Strawberries tend to turn to alcohol quickly because of their high-sugar content.

This recipe yields 1 quart of fruit or vegetable kvass.

Ingredients

1 cup coarsely chopped fruit or berries, vegetables, or a combination
Garlic cloves and/or ginger root, grated or minced (as desired)
½ cup whey from yogurt or kefir

Instructions

1. Place all ingredients in a wide-mouth quart jar. Fill jar with pure spring or filtered water to the shoulder, leaving about 2 inches of space between the top of the liquid and the lid. Cap tightly.

2. Leave on counter at room temperature for 2–3 days, or until the lid becomes taut under the pressure of your finger. Store in the refrigerator. To drink, pour out a serving and enjoy it straight, or dilute with equal parts water or mineral water.

3. To enjoy a second batch, choose one of the options below:

   Begin from scratch option: Replenish jar with more water after you pour out each serving and place jar back into the refrigerator. When the fruit is pale, begin again from scratch. Note: This will result in diluting the batch a bit every time.

   Easy second batch option: Rather than replenish the water every time you pour out a serving, wait until only about a quarter of the kvass remains. Fill jar back up to the shoulder with pure water, cap tightly, and leave on the counter for 2–3 days, or until the lid is taut. Enjoy batch #2 from the same fruits or vegetables! After you finish the second batch, discard the fruits or vegetables and start a new batch from the recipe.

Beet Kvass

Beet kvass is a liver tonic and blood cleanser. Tonics are especially healing to the body—they help "tone" a specific organ or organ systems. For example, beet kvass tones the liver and helps purify the blood.

However, drinking too much at once can provoke a detoxification reaction (diarrhea, cramping, vomiting in the extreme). When you first start drinking beet kvass, I suggest drinking 1 teaspoon of beet kvass, diluted with an equal amount of water, once a day for several days. Move on to a single (1 oz.) serving of beet kvass, diluted with an equal amount of water, once a day for several days. Eventually, you will work your way up to two (4 oz.) servings of diluted beet kvass per day, which is the daily maximum recommended amount.

This recipe yields 2 quarts of beet kvass.

Ingredients

1 medium organic beet, sliced fine (do not grate or the beets will turn to alcohol)
1–2 tablespoons sea salt
5 cloves garlic, peeled
1 cup whey (optional, see note below)

1 teaspoon grated ginger (optional)
Pure water

No whey option: If you omit the whey, increase salt to 2 tablespoons

Instructions

1. Place all ingredients in a wide-mouth 2-quart jar with a 2-piece lid. Fill jar with pure spring or filtered water to the shoulder, leaving about 2 inches between the ferment and the lid. Cap tightly.
2. Leave on counter at room temperature for 2–5 days, or until lid becomes taut under the pressure of your finger. Store in the refrigerator. To drink, pour out a serving and enjoy it straight, or dilute with equal parts water or mineral water.
3. To enjoy a second batch, choose one of the options below:

   Begin from scratch option: Replenish jar with more water after you pour out each serving and place jar back into the refrigerator. When the beet is pale, begin again from scratch. Note: This will result in diluting the batch a bit every time.

   Easy second batch option: Rather than replenish the water every time you pour out a serving, wait until only about a quarter of the beet kvass remains. Fill jar back up to the shoulder with pure water, cap tightly, and leave on counter for 2–3 days, or until the lid is taut. Enjoy batch #2 from the same beets! After you finish the second batch, discard the beets and start a new batch from the recipe.

Lacto-Fermented Vegetables

Because vegetables can be injurious to the gut lining, lacto-fermented vegetables do not make their debut until Stage 3 of the Intro diet. During the first two stages of the Intro, you stick with lacto-fermented tonics or beverages, or the juice of ferments (what I call "bug juice").

You can ferment nearly any vegetable you please, and I encourage you to try your hand at as many of them as you like, as well as various starters. You will eat vegetable ferments both in the Intro and the Full GAPS diet (and beyond). They are delicious and nutritious, so you should consider them part of a healthy diet even after your gut is healed and sealed.

The following Vegetable Medley recipe is specific to GAPS, and the sauerkraut is an old faithful. Enjoy!

Vegetable Medley

This medley is from *Gut and Psychology Syndrome* by Dr. Natasha Campbell-McBride. It is great for the Intro because of the amount of liquid (aka ferment juice) it contains. You may drink the ferment juice early on in the Intro, and when you are ready for Stage 3, you may eat the fermented vegetables. Simply follow the instructions to keep your medley going.

The recipe calls for whey from kefir (page 86). After you have made your first batch, you may wish to change the source of the whey. By switching the whey, you switch the lactobacilli. In doing so, you benefit from a wider variety of microbes with which to repopulate your gut flora.

Feel free to double this recipe. You may also add a variety of vegetables: cauliflower, sliced carrot, Brussels sprouts, broccoli, and so on. You can keep the vegetable medley going forever!

This recipe yields 2 quarts.

Ingredients

½ cabbage, roughly cut into bite-sized pieces
1 medium beet, cut into bite-sized pieces
½ teaspoon dill seeds or 1 tablespoon fresh dill, chopped
4–5 garlic cloves, peeled and chopped
1 tablespoon sea salt
½ cup kefir whey

Instructions

1. Fill a wide-mouth 2-quart wide-mouth jar halfway with vegetables. Add salt and kefir whey. Add pure spring or filtered water to the shoulder, leaving about 2 inches of space between the top of the liquid and the lid. You may cover the vegetables with cabbage leaves or use fermentation weights to keep the vegetables submerged under the brine. Cap tightly.

2. Leave on counter and ferment at room temperature for 1–2 weeks, or until the lid becomes taut under the pressure of your finger. Move jar to refrigerator. You may now start eating the vegetables.

3. To enjoy a second batch, when brine and vegetables start getting low, add fresh cabbage, beet, garlic, and some salt. Top with water and let ferment at room temperature again for another 1–2 weeks.

4. Repeat step 3. As previously stated, this can be your "forever ferment."

Sauerkraut

It is important that you do not over-pack the cabbage in this recipe because it will expand as it ferments. If you leave enough room between the top of the cabbage and the lid (about 2 inches), your jar will not leak on your counter, nor will it explode or bow with the pressure of fermentation. Also, please do not "burp" your ferments. Remember, fermentation is an anaerobic process—lactobacilli do not like oxygen.

Sauerkraut will keep for a few months after opening. But it only gets better with age, so try to wait a while before you dig in!

This recipe yields one quart of sauerkraut.

Ingredients

1 medium cabbage (any color or type that you prefer)
1 tablespoon caraway seeds (optional)
1 tablespoon sea salt
4 tablespoons whey (optional, see note below)

Optional add-ins: peeled, diced apples, finely grated carrots, green onions, or any other vegetables you would like to add

No whey option: If you omit the whey, increase salt to 2 tablespoons

Instructions

1. Using a very sharp knife or mandolin, shred cabbage very fine. (If you wish, retain an outer leaf of the cabbage to cover the kraut.) Place shredded cabbage in a large, stainless steel bowl.

2. Add all other ingredients to bowl. Pound mixture with a meat pounder or massage between your clean hands for 10 minutes. The cabbage will become limp and very bright in color as the water is drawn out of the leaves. Alternatively, you may sprinkle the cabbage with the salt, cover with a plate, and let sit on the counter for up to 6 hours or so. The salt will do the work for you, drawing out the water from the cabbage and into the bowl.

3. Place mixture and all of the liquid in a wide-mouth quart jar, leaving 1–2 inches of space from the top. Be sure cabbage is submerged below the brine. You may wish to cover the cabbage with cabbage leaves, or use fermentation weights to keep the kraut submerged under the brine. (The liquid should always cover the ingredient you are lacto-fermenting). Cap with lid and seal tightly.

4. Leave on counter at room temperature a minimum of 5–7 days, or until the lid

becomes taut under the pressure of your finger. (If you prefer a milder sauerkraut, you may leave it for 2 weeks or more.)

5. Place in cold storage, about 40°F (such as the top shelf of your refrigerator or a root cellar).

Frequently Asked Questions

10

I am lactose intolerant. Can I eat lacto-fermented foods?

Though it is easy to associate *lactose* with *lacto-ferment*, they do not mean the same thing. "Lacto-fermented" foods are simply foods made from lactic-acid producing bacteria (lactobacilli). In fact, you do not need to use dairy at all to lacto-ferment a food, though when you use whey as a starter, it lends valuable bacteria and loads the deck in favor of the gut good guys.

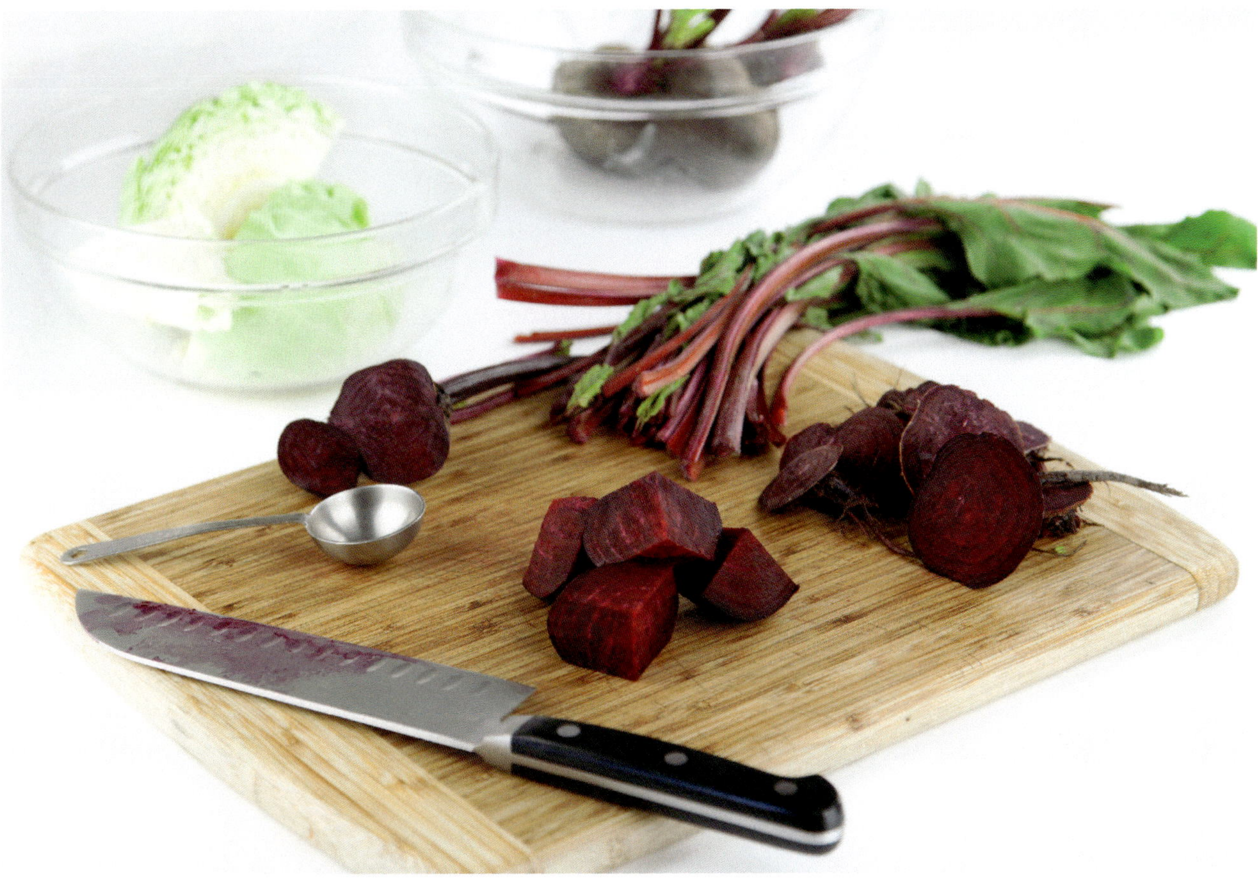

Hey! I see some white spots on the top of my ferment. What are they, and is my ferment still safe to eat?

Those white spots are an overgrowth of what is called "kahm yeast." They can form on your ferment if there is not enough salt in the brine, if the temperature is too warm, if there is too much oxygen in the ferment, or if the ferment is contaminated during preparation. In *Nourishing Traditions*, Sally Fallon suggests you simply scrape off and discard the white spots. You may then continue eating the ferment.

Why are my vegetables slimy?

Sometimes you may find a layer of slime on the top of the vegetables in your ferment. You may even find the vegetables themselves are slimy. Once again, yeast is the culprit! Scrape off and discard. The ferment is still safe to eat.

What about those black, green, pink, or red fuzzy spots?

Those spots are mold, but you may still have good fermented vegetables below the brine. Scrape off and discard. Wait a few moments, then smell the ferment. If the ferment smells okay, it should be okay to eat. But always listen to your gut! ***As always, if you don't feel comfortable eating the ferment, throw it out and start over***.

What if my ferment smells bad?

Your nose knows! If ever a ferment smells "off" to you, discard it.

My ferments leaked all over the counter! What happened, and what can I do to keep it from happening again?

If your ferments leak on the counter, you did not leave enough space between the ingredients and the top of the jar. Remember, vegetables need enough space to expand during fermentation. If you leave two inches or so of space, the ferment will not leak.

Does it matter what size I cut my vegetables?

In general, the smaller the vegetables, the faster they will ferment. It is usually a good idea to cut them bite size. However, when it comes to beets, be mindful of how small you cut them. Beets are high in sugar, so if you cut them too small, your ferment may turn to alcohol.

Can I use tap water to ferment with a brine?

No! I never recommended tap water for lacto-fermentation. Tap water is full of chemicals that are designed to kill microbes, which means they can also kill your gut good guys. The best option for fermentation is spring or filtered water.

Can I ferment in direct sunlight?

No! While you can keep your ferments on the counter, leaving jars in direct sunlight can cook your microbes. Explosions can ensue.

Can I ferment my jars near the microwave?

Only if you never use it. We are trying to grow lactobacilli. Who knows what microwaves will do to them.

Why is kombucha not included in this book?

Kombucha is not a lacto-ferment. It is a very different process, aerobic, even. Making kombucha involves a symbiotic colony of bacteria and yeast (SCOBY). Although it is a tonic, kombucha is not officially part of the GAPS diet. It can be problematic for those with candida overgrowth.

Sources

The Great and Varied Benefits of Lacto-Fermentation

Tamang, J.P., Shin, D. Jung, S. and Chae, S. "Functional Properties of Microorganisms in Fermented Foods." Frontiers in Microbiology, April 26, 2016.

Lacto-Fermentation vs. Canning Chart

"CFI Fact Sheet: Canning Food Safely." Center for Foodborne Illness Research and Prevention.

LaBorde, L., and Zepp, M. "Let's Preserve: Basics of Home Canning." Penn State Extension, Penn State College of Agricultural Sciences, 2013.

"How Canning Preserves Food." Clemson University Department of Food, Nutrition, and Packaging Science, 2012.

Frei, R., Akdis, M., and O'Mahony, L. "Prebiotics, Probiotics, Synbiotics, and the Immune System: Experimental Data and Clinical Evidence." Current Opinion in Gastroenterology, 31(2):153–158, March 2015.

Wollowski, I., Rechkemmer, G., and Pool-Zobel, B.L. "Protective Role of Probiotics and Prebiotics in Colon Cancer." American Journal of Clinical Nutrition, 73(2 Suppl):451S–455S, February 2001.

Ouwehand, A.C., Salminen, S., and Isolauri, E. "Probiotics: An Overview of Beneficial Effects." Antonie Van Leeuwenhoek, 82(1–4):279–289, August 2002.

Reid, G., Jass, J., Sebulsky, M.T., and McCormick, J.K. "Potential Uses of Probiotics in Clinical Practice." Clinical Microbiology Reviews, 16(4):658–672, October 2003.

Yakovlieva, M., Tacheva, T., Mihaylova, S., Tropcheva, R., Trifonova, K., Tolekova, A., Danova, S., Vlaykova, T. "Influence of Lactobacillus Brevis 15 and Lactobacillus Plantarum 13 on Blood Glucose and Body Weight in Rats After High-Fructose Diet." Beneficial Microbes, 6(4):505–512, 2015.

Section X | Seeds (Nuts, Seeds, Beans, and Grains)

Foreword

> Monica Corrado has done a wonderful job of explaining how to cook and prepare nuts, seeds, and legumes in this book. These foods require proper preparation in order to make them digestible and derive maximum nutrition from them. I believe that all human beings have a limited ability to digest these foods and should know how to handle them. But it is particularly important for people with any digestive problems, such as those on the GAPS diet. I would like to thank Monica for doing this work! She has written this book with her usual practical no-nonsense approach and her lovely sense of humor. I highly recommend this book to everyone on GAPS, and to any other person who would like to use nuts, seeds and legumes in their diet.
>
> —Dr. Natasha Campbell-McBride

Seeds (Nuts, Seeds, Beans, and Grains)

Introduction

In this section we will dive into nuts, seeds, beans, and, to a lesser extent, grains. I believe that learning how to work with these ingredients is second only to understanding the crucial role that Meat Stock and Bone Broth both play in the GAPS nutritional protocol.

Why? Because like Meat Stock and Bone Broth, the role of nuts, seeds, and beans in the GAPS diet is also misunderstood. For starters, did you know that all of these are, well, seeds? And that many of us are not aware of the fact that we need to prepare seeds properly to make them more digestible? Not doing so can lead to digestive distress, bloating, and cramping—and even mineral deficiencies that cause further injury.

Where do nuts, seeds, and beans fit in the GAPS diet? Read on to find out. Learn what they are. Why you should eat them. When you should eat them. And, most of all, how to apply the time-honored techniques that unlock their nutrients and make them available to your body. By the time you reach the end of this section, I hope to make it clear how important these techniques are.

For the purposes of the GAPS diet, where we are encouraging a healing process by lightening some of the burden off the digestion process, we will spend most of this section on nuts and seeds. But you will also find important techniques for working with the few specific beans allowed on the GAPS diet.

There are no grains on GAPS at all, until you are ready to go off GAPS and start the Transition Diet. (Yes, people do!) And because you will one day as well, I've included a bonus chapter on working with grains. Refer to those techniques when you are ready.

Happy reading!

Seeds (Nuts, Seeds, Beans, and Grains)

What Are Nuts, Seeds, Beans, and Grains?

1

There are many, many types of seeds on the planet, but for culinary, horticultural, and agricultural purposes, it is useful to place various types of seeds into separate categories: nuts, seeds, beans, and grains.

That's right. Every nut, every grain, and every bean is a SEED. I say this to the students in my Cooking for Well-Being classes over and over again, until it becomes ingrained their memories.

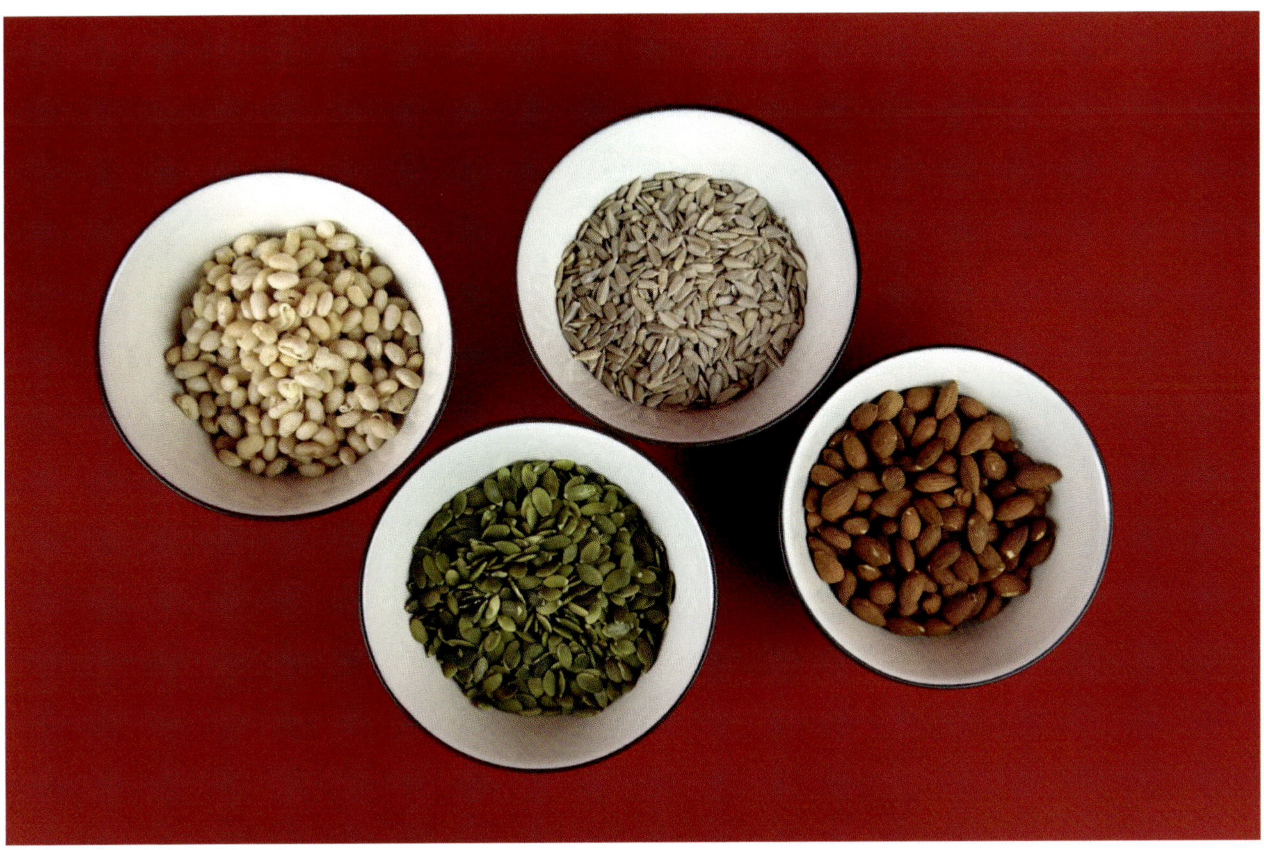

Read it again. And again. That one sentence holds the clue as to why every traditional society the world over does something to nuts and seeds (and beans and grains) before cooking and eating them.

To understand why, you only need to understand two things: First, no matter what category we place them in, all seeds are the means by which a plant procreates, and they would rather procreate than be eaten. Second, to keep from being eaten, seeds evolved to be hard on our digestive system.

In fact, you may be surprised to learn that nuts, seeds, beans, and grains are the number one hardest thing for the human body to digest. This is another thing I say often to my students, much to their disbelief. Yes, 'tis true. Perhaps you thought it was that grass-fed T-bone steak, but the incisors in your mouth and the HCl in your stomach make easy work of meat.

Plants are a different story. They do not want the seeds of their progeny destroyed—they want them to become new plants, and those new plants want to procreate. That is why seeds evolved to withstand digestion by you, me, and every other human, animal, or fowl that endeavors to eat them.

Somewhere along the way, however, humans learned how to unlock these nutritional powerhouses by applying predigestion techniques—that is, soaking, sprouting, and fermenting—before eating them. And for the benefits we derive in turn, this bit of extra work is a small price to pay!

It is true that if your digestive system is intact, you should have little problem digesting some seeds, such as sesame seeds. And you can always help your digestive system along simply by chewing. Remember your mother telling you to chew your food? As you chew, your mouth soaks your food, increasing your ability to break it down and absorb its nutrients. The mechanical act of chewing, along with good saliva enzymes, helps predigest some starches and fats enough to begin the digestion process before the stomach has its turn. So be wise and listen to your mother: don't forget to chew!

However, for the reasons I mention above, eating most nuts and seeds in their raw state is not optimal, and this is especially true if you have a compromised gut. That is why we need to do a little bit more in order to avoid the risk of digestive distress. Enter GAPS. This healing protocol was specifically designed to encourage healing by lightening some of the burden off the digestion process. That is exactly what predigestion techniques are for—and, of course, what this section is all about!

Seeds (Nuts, Seeds, Beans, and Grains)

The Role of Nuts and Seeds in the GAPS Diet

2

Nuts and seeds play several important roles in the GAPS diet. For one, you can use them to diversify your menu. By the time you get to Stage 3 of the Intro, you may be missing some baked goods and looking forward to introducing them back into your diet. For example, in Stage 3, you may introduce nuts and seeds as Nut or Seed Butter Pancakes. And in Stage 4, you may introduce nut or seed flour as Basic Bread. Or, if you cannot tolerate nuts or seeds, you may use cooked and fermented white navy bean flour instead. Once you tolerate Basic Bread, you may even introduce muffins and cakes.

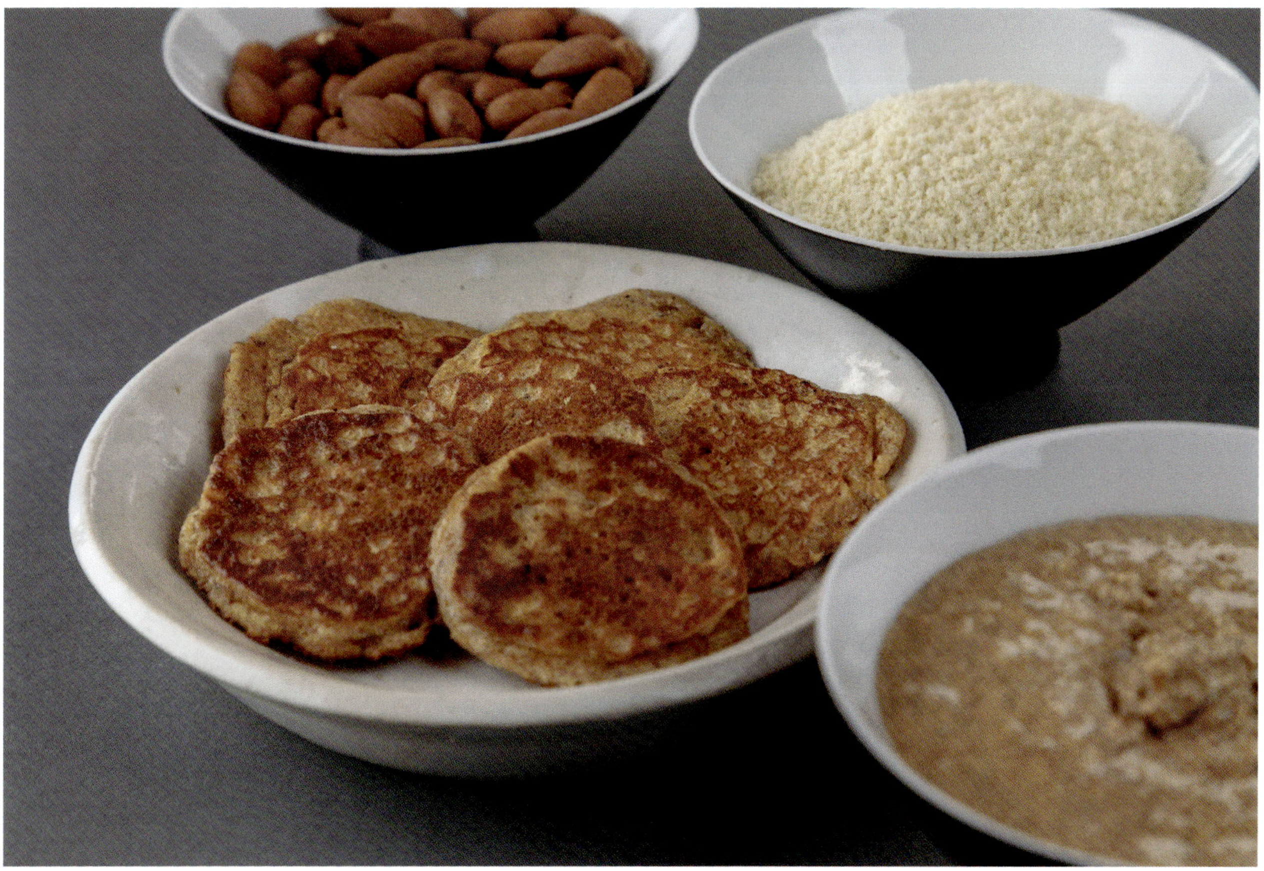

Please note, however, that with the exception of the Nut or Seed Butter Pancakes in Stage 3, baked goods are *meant to be treats* for occasional consumption. They are, after all, a challenge for the digestive system, so do not be in a rush to introduce them. And do not be surprised if they set off symptoms you thought were gone for good! Slow and steady when it comes to healing with the GAPS diet. Remember, it took you a while to get into this state of dis-ease, and it will take time to remedy it.

Another important role that nuts and seeds play in the GAPS diet has to do with the fiber they contain. In addition to neutralizing the antinutrients in nuts and seeds, those with compromised guts must address yet another digestive challenge. Nuts and seeds themselves—how they are packaged, if you will—are high in fiber, which is not allowed during the beginning stages of the Intro diet. Early on, fiber can act as sandpaper on the damaged intestinal walls (not a pretty image, I know), causing further injury.

However, as you progress in the Intro, you will gradually introduce more and more challenging foods into your diet. Once you get to Stage 3 and introduce nuts and seeds, you will find that the fiber they contain acts as a sort of test to help measure the level of healing in your digestive system. If it turns out that you cannot tolerate the fiber, even after pulverizing nuts or seeds into butter or flour, you are not yet ready to introduce nuts and seeds.

When you are ready to introduce baked goods in Stage 3 of the Intro, you can help set yourself up for success by keeping these two things in mind:

1. You must neutralize the antinutrients in the nuts and seeds by soaking, sprouting, and/or fermenting them.
2. You must avoid causing yourself harm or injury by reducing the fiber content in nuts and seeds. Pulverizing them into nut or seed butter or making them into nut or seed flour helps break the fiber down ahead of time.

Finally, nuts and seeds play a third important role in the GAPS diet by providing alternative sources of fat and protein, as you can see from the chart below.

Percentage of Carbohydrates, Protein, and Fat in Some Nuts and Seeds

	Carbohydrate	Protein	Fat
Almonds	15	13	72
Brazil nuts	14.5	14.5	70
Cashews	22	11.5	66.5
Pecans	8	5	87
Pumpkin seeds	13	16	71
Sunflower seeds	17	11.5	71.5
Walnuts	8.5	8	83.5

Seeds (Nuts, Seeds, Beans, and Grains)

Nuts or Seeds? And Which Nuts or Seeds?

3

Nuts and seeds present a challenge to most digestive systems—even healthy ones—because they are all protected by natural chemical compounds known as antinutrients. While antinutrients are a normal component of food and play a critical role in the life of the seed, they are hard to digest. For those on the GAPS healing protocol, they must be neutralized or broken down before eating. Traditional preparation methods for neutralizing the antinutrients in most nuts and seeds involve some form of soaking, sprouting, fermenting, and cooking, all of which are covered in later chapters. But before you even get to the techniques, the first step is knowing what kind of nuts and seeds to purchase.

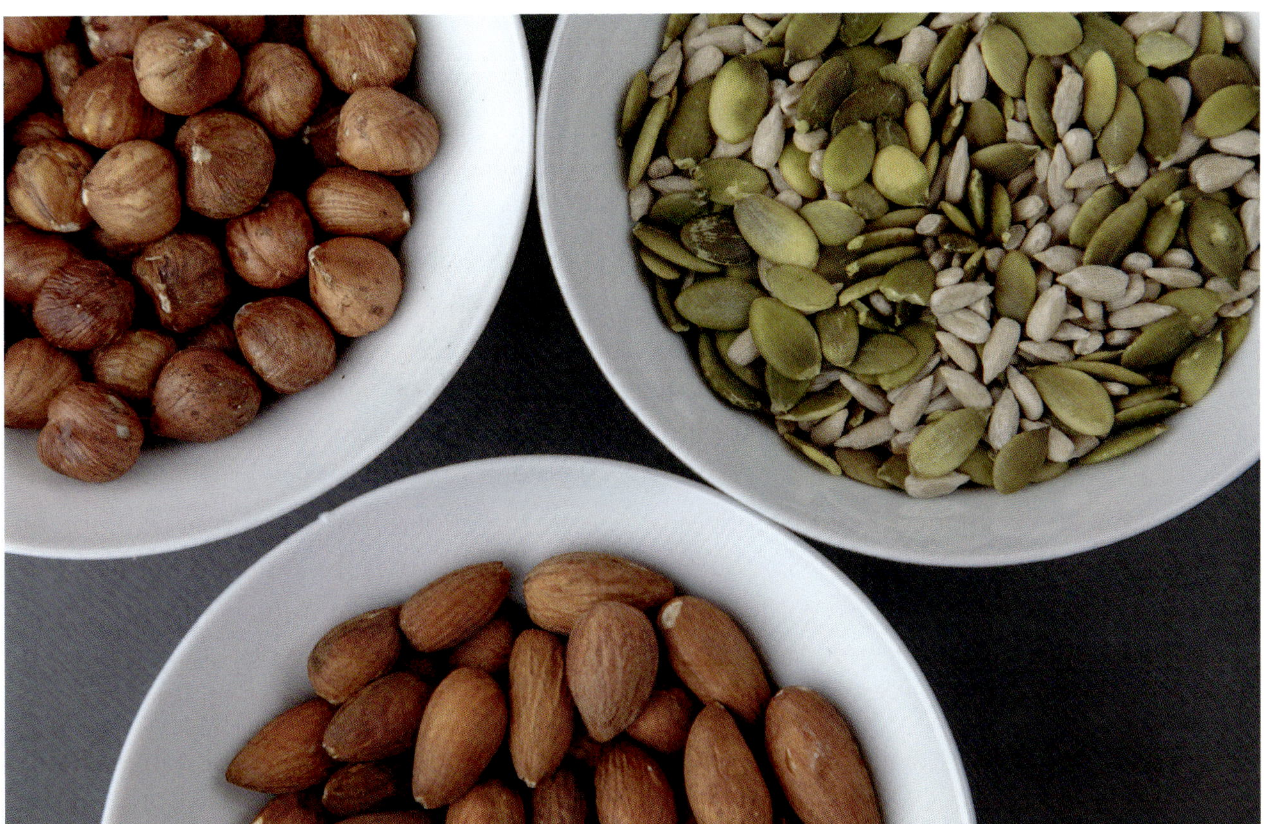

Important Notes on Purchasing Nuts and Seeds

Organic: Purchase only organic nuts and seeds. Organic foods cannot be irradiated. If organic is not available, make sure the nuts and seeds you do purchase have not been irradiated because this decreases their nutrient value and kills important enzymes. If the package has a label, look for the statements "Treated with radiation" or "Treated by irradiation." Bulk food bins are required by the FDA to have a label next to the sale container.

> Irradiated legumes, nuts, grains, and seeds usually will not sprout—but who would want to eat them anyway?

Raw and intact: Purchase nuts and seeds in their raw state, and still in their shells if possible. You want all the goodness of the nut or seed intact, just as Mother Nature intended. Once that protective shell is opened or broken, the nut or seed is exposed to heat, light, and oxygen. Why is that bad? Because all nuts and seeds contain a good amount of fat, and fat goes rancid when exposed to these elements. To minimize the possibility of exposure and rancidity, do not remove the shells until right before you use them. If you must purchase shelled nuts or seeds, get them in small batches and keep them well sealed in the refrigerator or freezer. Raw, of course, excludes all nuts or seeds that have been roasted, salted, or coated in any way, including those coated with cottonseed oil, canola oil, soy oil, or any other oil. These oils are all probably rancid themselves.

Beware of bulk bins: While bulk bins of shelled nuts or nut flour seem inexpensive at first glance, chances are high that their contents have been exposed to light and air for a good period of time. The probability of rancidity depends on the amount and type of fat in the nut or seed, especially if it is high in good fats. In general, nuts and seeds rich in polyunsaturated fats go rancid more quickly than those rich in saturated fats. Almonds, pecans, cashews, and macadamia nuts are all high in stable oleic acid. Walnuts, however, contain large amounts of triple unsaturated linolenic acid, which is unstable and goes rancid quickly. See *Nourishing Traditions* (p. 513) by Sally Fallon Morell to learn more.

Nuts High in Polyunsaturated Fats

	Grams of fat per 100 gm serving
Walnuts	47
Pine nuts	34
Sunflower seeds	23
Sesame seeds	22
Pecans	22
Brazil nuts	21
Pumpkin seeds	21

Nuts vs. seeds: Nuts are generally more difficult to digest than seeds. If your digestive system is challenged, it is probably best to start with seeds. Either way, be sure to apply one of the predigestion techniques outlined in chapter 9 before you eat any nut or seed.

Which nuts? All nuts are allowed on the GAPS diet. Almonds are often listed as the nut of choice in recipes, but walnuts, almonds, Brazil nuts, pecans, hazelnuts, and cashews are all interchangeable. Even peanuts, which are technically legumes, are allowed on GAPS.

What about cashews? Cashews are classified as seeds of the cashew apple rather than nuts. In fact, cashews (Anacardium occidentale) are in the same family as poison ivy and poison sumac. Because their shells contain a highly toxic oil, they cannot be sold in their shells.

In order to access the nut, neutralize the toxic oil, and make them safe to eat, cashews go through four stages of processing during harvesting: steam roasting, shell cutting, peeling, and grading. By the end, the cashews have been cooked and their enzymes have been destroyed. That means "raw" cashews are not really raw!

Also, because they undergo so many processes just to make them edible, cashews are more delicate and take less time to soak or ferment than other nuts and seeds.

> In addition to enzyme inhibitors, phytates, and lectins, almonds and cashews are also high in oxalic acid (or oxalates). Oxalic acid can also bind with minerals such as calcium, magnesium, iron, sodium, and potassium, blocking their absorption in the digestive tract. You can reduce the amount of oxalic acid in almonds or cashews by—you guessed it—soaking, sprouting, or fermenting them.

Which seeds? Sunflower seeds and pumpkin seeds are often called for in GAPS recipes. Other seeds are simply too small for applying a predigestion technique, not to mention grinding into flour for baking. The exception is sesame seed butter (tahini). Sesame seeds are chock-full of nutrients, and you do not need to do any soaking, sprouting, or fermenting to unlock them.

The bean alternative: If you cannot tolerate nuts or seeds, you may try fermented white navy beans for baking instead. However, be warned: this is a very involved process, and some of us do not want to eat a baked good so badly that we are willing to go through it.

Options for storage: To prevent rancidity, it is important to store shelled nuts (those that have been taken out of their shells) and seeds at room temperature in an airtight container. Keep them in a cool, dark place, where they will last about a month. Store glass jars in a pantry or cupboard. However, the best way to store shelled nuts or seeds is in the refrigerator or freezer. If refrigerated, they should last up to six months. If frozen, up to a year. Mark your nut containers with dates so you can keep track and use them before the end of the storage time. Nuts and seeds are expensive! You don't want to lose them because you can't remember when you put them into cold storage.

Seeds (Nuts, Seeds, Beans, and Grains)

Introducing Nuts, Seeds, and Beans

4

You do not introduce nuts and seeds until Stage 3 of the Intro diet, after you have successfully experienced some healing in your gut. As always in the GAPS healing protocol, when you introduce a new food, you introduce it in the form that is easiest on your digestive system. Please note that the introduction of nuts or seeds too early can set your healing back. Dr. Natasha suggests that people introduce nuts and seeds very slowly, and to watch for the reoccurrence of symptoms with their introduction.

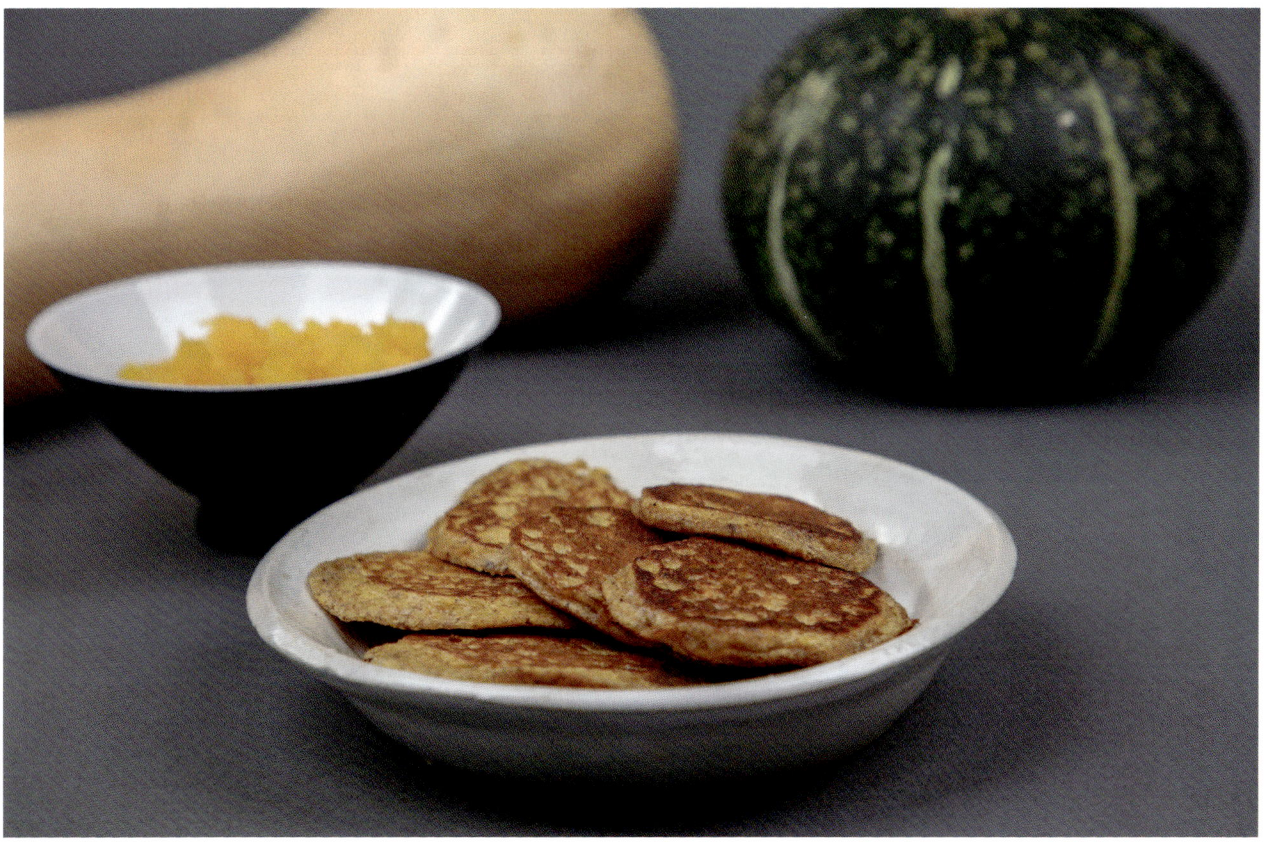

The easiest way to digest nuts and seeds is to make them into nut or seed butter, which you can then use to make the Nut or Seed Butter Pancakes (chapter 10). To introduce nuts or seeds as butter, you grind them into a paste until they are pulverized and spreadable, like, well…butter. Because the fiber is broken down in the food processor in the process, nut and seed butters are easiest on the digestive system and pose less of a threat to the gut lining.

However, nut and seed butters present another digestive challenge: fat. Because they are high in fat, they can stress the liver and gallbladder. A sign that you are eating more nut or seed butter than your body can handle is nausea. If you experience this, take a few days off. Afterwards, reintroduce the butter in a very small amount, perhaps a teaspoon or so, and slowly increase as tolerated. To help your liver and gallbladder handle the additional fat, you may want to try increasing the amount of beet kvass in your diet. (For the recipe and details, see Section IX: Lacto-Fermentation.)

After your body can tolerate nut or seed butter, you gradually introduce nuts and seeds in forms that are progressively more challenging to digest (see chart on following page). Nut and seed flours are a little more challenging for the digestive system than butters, so you will wait until Stage 5 to introduce them as Basic Bread and other baked goods.

Finally, we come to whole nuts or seeds. Because of their fibrous nature, you do not introduce these until after your gut has been healed and sealed—that is, *after* you have completed all six stages of the Intro and have graduated to the Full GAPS diet. Healing and sealing of the gut lining takes place while you are on the Intro diet. The goal of following the Full GAPS diet for two years after the Intro is to continue to strengthen your digestive system and prevent further injury.

Ultimately, how easy it is for you to digest nuts and seeds depends on several factors, especially the predigestion technique you use to neutralize the antinutrients: soaking, sprouting, and/or fermenting, and the form of preparation you choose: nut or seed butter (Stage 3) or flour (Stage 5), or as whole nuts or seeds (Full GAPS).

Scale of Digestibility

Hardest to digest →				*Easiest to digest*
Whole nuts and seeds:				
Raw *(no preparation)*	Soaked	Sprouted	Fermented	Soaked or sprouted, then fermented
Nut or seed flour made from:				
Raw nuts or seeds *(no preparation)*	Soaked nuts or seeds	Sprouted nuts or seeds	Fermented nuts or seeds	Flour that is fermented
Nut or seed butter made from:				
Raw nuts or seeds *(no preparation)*	Soaked nuts or seeds	Sprouted nuts or seeds	Fermented nuts or seeds	

Let's sum it up: if nuts and seeds cause digestive distress when you introduce them into your diet, you must do two things in order to make them easy on your digestive system and access their nutrients. As the Scale of Digestibility shows, you must:

1. Form of nut or seed: Introduce nuts and seeds in a form that is easiest to digest before moving on to progressively more challenging forms. The top line of the **Scale of Digestibility** shows that nut or seed butter is easiest to digest, while nut or seed flour is easier than whole nuts or seeds.

2. Preparation technique: Neutralize the antinutrients with a predigestion process. As the bottom line in the **Scale of Digestibility** illustrates, sprouting is better than soaking, fermenting is better than sprouting, the best predigestion process of all is to either soak or sprout, and then ferment.

As you can see above, butter made from nuts or seeds that you soak or sprout and then ferment are easiest on the digestive system. Eating raw, whole nuts or seeds is the most difficult.

A Small Amount Is a Small Amount

As always, introduce a small amount at a time, and introduce that same small amount every day for three to five days before you increase the amount. As I noted in Section VIII: Culturing Dairy, "A small amount is a small amount. It may be what fits on the head of a pin." In the case of Nut or Seed Butter Pancakes, it may be as little as one small bite.

When eating Nut or Seed Butter Pancakes, Basic Bread or other baked goods, or a handful of nuts as a snack, if at any point you experience digestive disturbance or the return of any symptoms, go back to the stage prior. Symptoms are unique to each individual and can be physical, mental, or emotional. Wait at least two weeks before trying to introduce the food again.

Because nuts and seeds do not want to be eaten, they are some of the hardest foods to introduce into the diet. You may experience a setback or the reappearance of symptoms. If this happens, do not be surprised. You are not in a race to complete the Intro. Taking it slow and steady will yield the deep healing you desire.

The Skin Sensitivity Test

What if you have a nut or seed allergy or sensitivity? If you suspect a sensitivity or allergy to a particular nut or seed, you should give yourself a Skin Sensitivity Test prior to introducing the nut or seed into your diet.

The Skin Sensitivity Test (or Sensitivity Test from here forward) tells you if you have a sensitivity to a certain food. It is very easy to do yourself at home, and far less expensive than an allergy test would be.

Take the Sensitivity Test if you have a known allergy or suspect a sensitivity to a food. Most individuals have reactions to protein, and nuts and seeds contain a good bit of protein. *Caution:* Do not introduce nuts or seeds to someone who has experienced a severe allergic reaction (anaphylaxis) to either.

How to do the Sensitivity Test: Be sure to test exactly what you will be eating. For example, if you will be eating nut butter you make at home, test for nut butter you make at home. If it is a certain brand of nut butter, test for that brand.

Place a drop of the food in question (mash solid food with a bit of water) on the inside of the wrist at bedtime. Let the drop dry on the skin (you may wish to cover it with a Band-Aid to keep it there). In the morning, check the spot. If there is a red reaction—what Dr. Natasha calls "an angry red spot"—avoid the food for a few weeks and then try again. If there is no reaction, you may introduce the food gradually, starting with a very small amount.

Remember, do not rush to introduce new foods. Watch to see if the new food triggers any symptoms—digestive, mental, or emotional. If you experience symptoms, either discontinue the food for two weeks or more and then do another test, or stay at the level where the symptom occurred until it passes. Once the symptom passes, you may very slowly increase the amount of the food that triggered the symptom.

Seeds (Nuts, Seeds, Beans, and Grains)

Nut and Seed Butters and Flours Are Not Created Equal

5

Why should you make your own nut or seed butter and flour? Because store-bought versions present some important challenges, as you will see below. As always, it is best to make your own.

Store-Bought Nut or Seed Butter

Commercially available nut and seed butters are usually made from raw or roasted nuts or seeds. Raw has the problems of

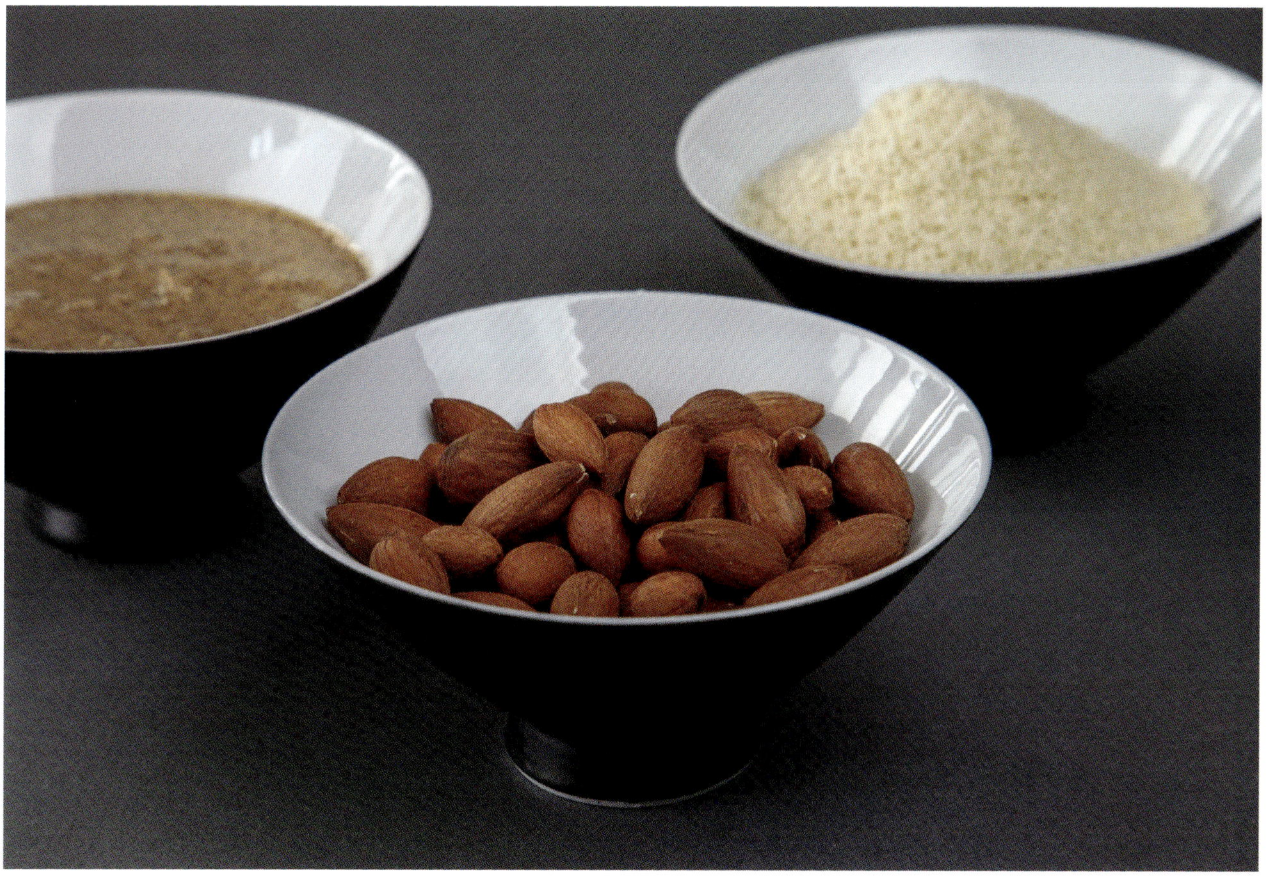

antinutrients, which must be neutralized by soaking, sprouting, or fermenting. This makes them easily digestible when your gut is compromised—and even after. Roasted has the problem of rancidity. Indeed, most store-bought nut or seed butters are rancid in the jar.

Over the past few years, some sprouted nut and seed butters have become available online and in stores, but these are very expensive. Making your own saves you money and rewards you with lots of easily digested protein and healthy fats—no antinutrients, no rancidity.

Options for Nut or Seed Butters

Here are your options for introducing store-bought or homemade nut or seed butters in Stage 3:

Not Recommended	Good	Best
Store-bought organic, roasted nut or seed butter	Store-bought organic, sprouted nut or seed butter	Store-bought nuts or seeds that you sprout, soak, or ferment, then use to make homemade nut butter

Nut or Seed Flour

Once nuts and seeds are ground into flour, the probability of rancidity increases dramatically. Flour stored in large bulk bins or plastic bags is even more susceptible to oxidation (which plays a huge role in rancidity).

Scale of Rancidity for Store-Bought Nut or Seed Flour

Most rancid →		***Least rancid***
Stored in bulk bins, under lights	Stored in clear plastic bags, under lights	Make your own, use immediately

Making your own is the most healthful option. Sprout or ferment your own organic nuts or seeds, then grind them into flour and use immediately.

> If a nut or seed is high in lauric acid, it will smell "soapy" as it goes rancid. An example is coconut oil.

Also keep in mind that some nuts go rancid more quickly than others. Nuts high in saturated fats (Brazil nuts, macadamias, almonds) tend to go rancid more slowly, while nuts high in polyunsaturated fats (walnuts, pecans, pine nuts) go rancid more quickly.

Options for Nut or Seed Flours

Here are your options for store-bought or homemade nut or seed flours for the Basic Bread in Stage 4:

Not Good	Better	Best	Best of the Best
Store-bought nut or seed flour *(may be rancid when purchased)*	Store-bought nut or seed flour, fermented before baking *(may be rancid when purchased)* Raw nuts you grind yourself *(no rancidity, antinutrients still present)* Raw nuts, soaked in salt and warm water for 7–18 hours, then ground into flour *(antinutrients neutralized, no rancidity)*	Raw nuts, sprouted, then ground into flour *(antinutrients neutralized, no rancidity)* Raw nuts, fermented, then ground into flour *(antinutrients neutralized, no rancidity)*	Raw nuts, soaked or sprouted, then fermented and ground into flour.

Seeds (Nuts, Seeds, Beans, and Grains)

Traditional Techniques to Neutralize Antinutrients

6

Soaking (with a deactivator or neutralizing agent), sprouting, and fermenting nuts and seeds are three methods that neutralize enzyme inhibitors and phytates, break down complex carbohydrates that cause gastric distress, and unlock nutrients so they are available to the body. This is especially important if your diet depends on nuts and seeds, as it prevents serious mineral deficiencies that can lead to bone loss.

As important as it is to apply at least one of these predigestion techniques for the reasons outlined above, they do not all arrive

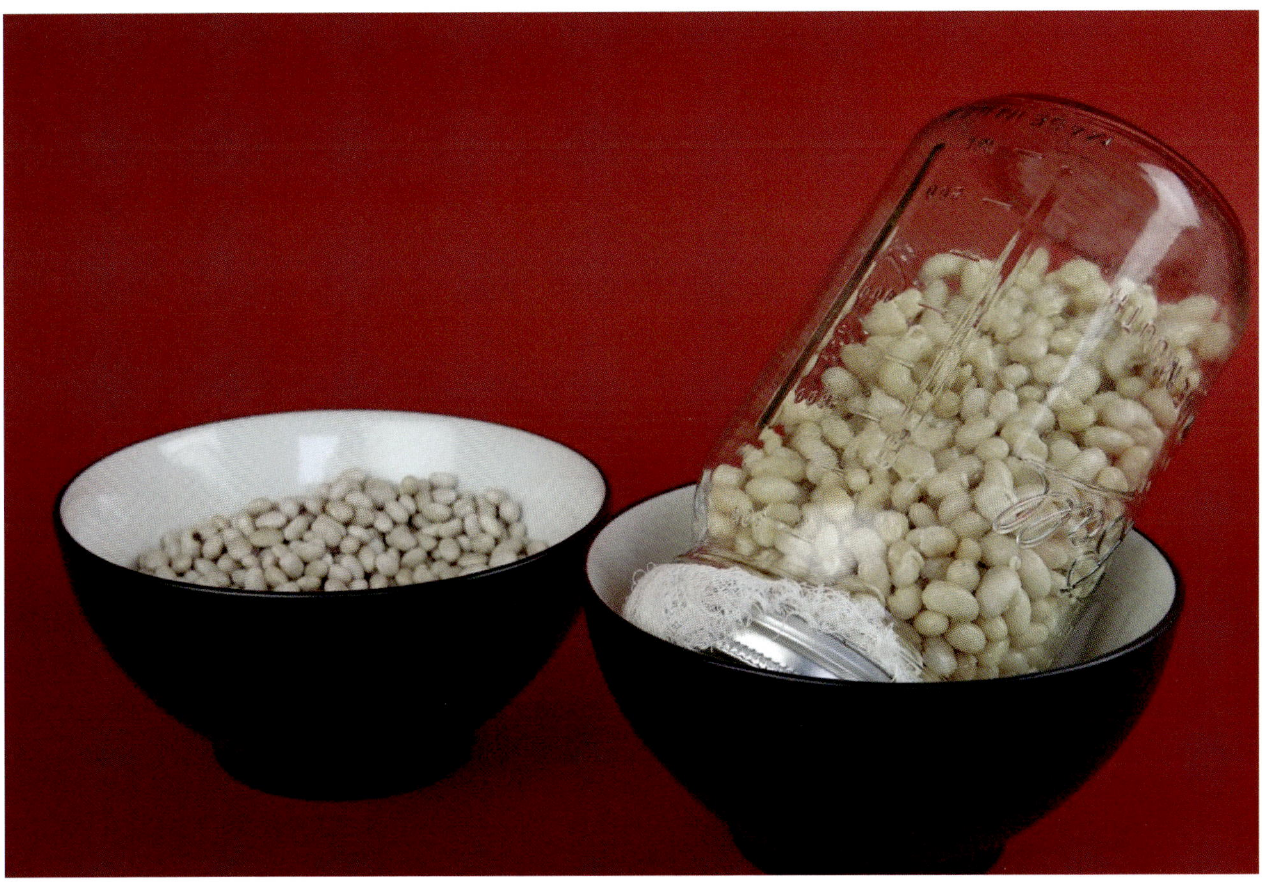

at the same end result. Sprouting works better than soaking, fermenting works better than sprouting, and a combination works the best of all, as this scale below shows:

Scale of Digestibility: Nuts and Seeds

Hardest to digest →					***Easiest to digest***
None *(Raw)*	Roast	Soak *(in saltwater)*	Sprout	Ferment	Soak or sprout, then ferment

Soaking Nuts and Seeds

To soak nuts and seeds, you need only three things: warm water, good salt, and time. For most nuts and seeds, you will need 7 hours minimum or 24 hours maximum of soak time. (The exception is cashews, which you should not soak for more than 6 hours.) You may dry soaked nuts and seeds using your oven or dehydrator and then make into nut or seed flour for use in baking.

If you soak, no need to sprout. If you sprout, no need to soak. But if you want the best predigestion technique of all, follow it up by fermenting.

When and how to use soaked nuts and seeds:

- Stage 3 of Intro: Pulverize into "butter" for use in Nut or Seed Butter Pancakes.
- Stage 4 of Intro: Make into flour for use in Nut or Seed Flour Pancakes and Basic Bread.
- Stage 6 of Intro and Full GAPS diet: Make into flour for use in other baked goods.

Sprouting Nuts and Seeds

Sprouting is another way to make nuts and seeds (and legumes) more nutrient dense and easier on the digestive system. It is also a simple way to neutralize the antinutrients and enzyme inhibitors. When you sprout, you are changing a seed into a plant.

Sprouting activates phytase, the enzyme that breaks down phytic acid. It also neutralizes enzyme inhibitors and reduces some of the carbohydrate content in nuts, seeds, beans, and grains, making them more like a vegetable and less like a starch.

Again, you may choose to soak or to sprout—no need to do both (though some people do).

When and how to use sprouted nuts and seeds:

- Stage 3 of Intro: Pulverize into "butter" for Nut or Seed Butter Pancakes.
- Stage 4 of Intro: Use as flour for Nut or Seed Flour Pancakes and Basic Bread.
- Stage 6 of Intro and Full GAPS diet: Make into flour for use in other baked goods.

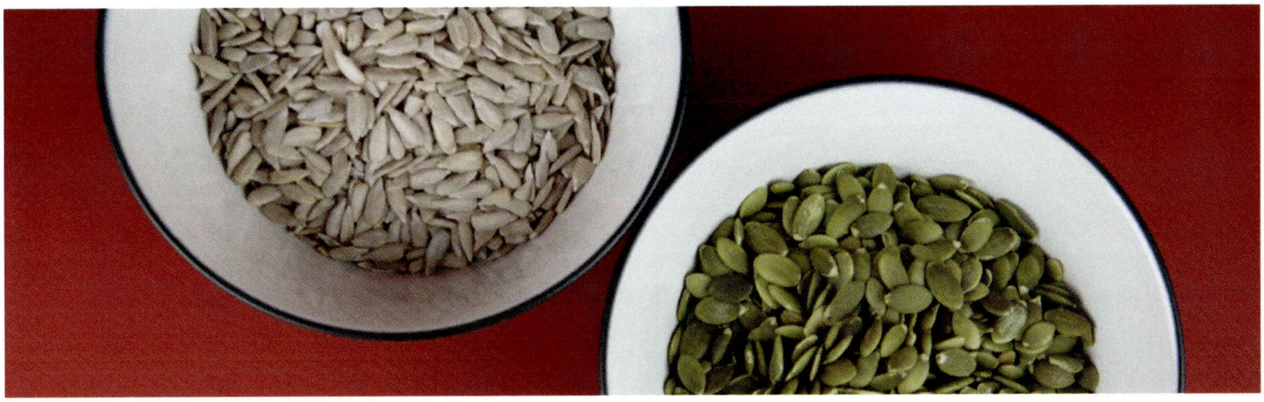

Fermenting Nuts or Seeds

As always, fermentation is the best predigestion technique. Let the microbes do the work for you! The more you can predigest your food before you eat it, the easier it is on your system and the more nutrients available to you.

You may ferment raw, soaked, or sprouted nuts and seeds. You may also ferment nut or seed flour for use in baking. In fact, taking the extra step of fermenting nut or seed flour is the gold standard of digestibility.

To ferment, you only need two things: whey or another fermentation starter and time. Recipes for making whey from kefir, yogurt, or raw milk are in Section VIII: Culturing Dairy.

When and how to use fermented nuts and seeds:

- Stage 3 of Intro: Pulverize into "butter" for Nut or Seed Butter Pancakes
- Stage 4 of Intro: Grind fermented nuts or seeds into flour and use in Nut or Seed Flour Pancakes and Basic Bread.
- Stage 6 of Intro and Full GAPS diet: Grind fermented nuts or seeds into flour and use in other baked goods.

You may also grind *raw* nuts or seeds into flour, and then ferment the flour. In other words, you may ferment the nuts and seeds and use them as above, or you may grind raw nuts or seeds first, and then ferment them.

Note: If you cannot tolerate nuts or seeds, you may use soaked or sprouted, fermented, and then cooked white navy beans for the Nut Butter Pancakes and Basic Bread instead.

What about beans, legumes, and grains? As you will see when you get to the techniques in chapter 9, you may sprout beans and legumes in the same way that you sprout nuts and seeds. However, soaking and fermenting them are different processes. And grains are different still. Grains are not even allowed until you have completed the Full GAPS diet (which takes about two years). But when you are on the Transition diet, certain sprouted grains are used (see chapter 12).

Seeds (Nuts, Seeds, Beans, and Grains)

Let's Talk About Beans and Legumes in the GAPS Diet

7

Yes, you may eat beans and other legumes in the GAPS diet. But only certain beans and legumes, and only at certain times. On the Intro diet, only white navy beans and peanuts are allowed (remember, peanuts are legumes). On the Full GAPS diet, you may add lentils and lima beans—but they first need to be soaked or sprouted, and then cooked. (The method for sprouting is the same as for nuts and seeds.)

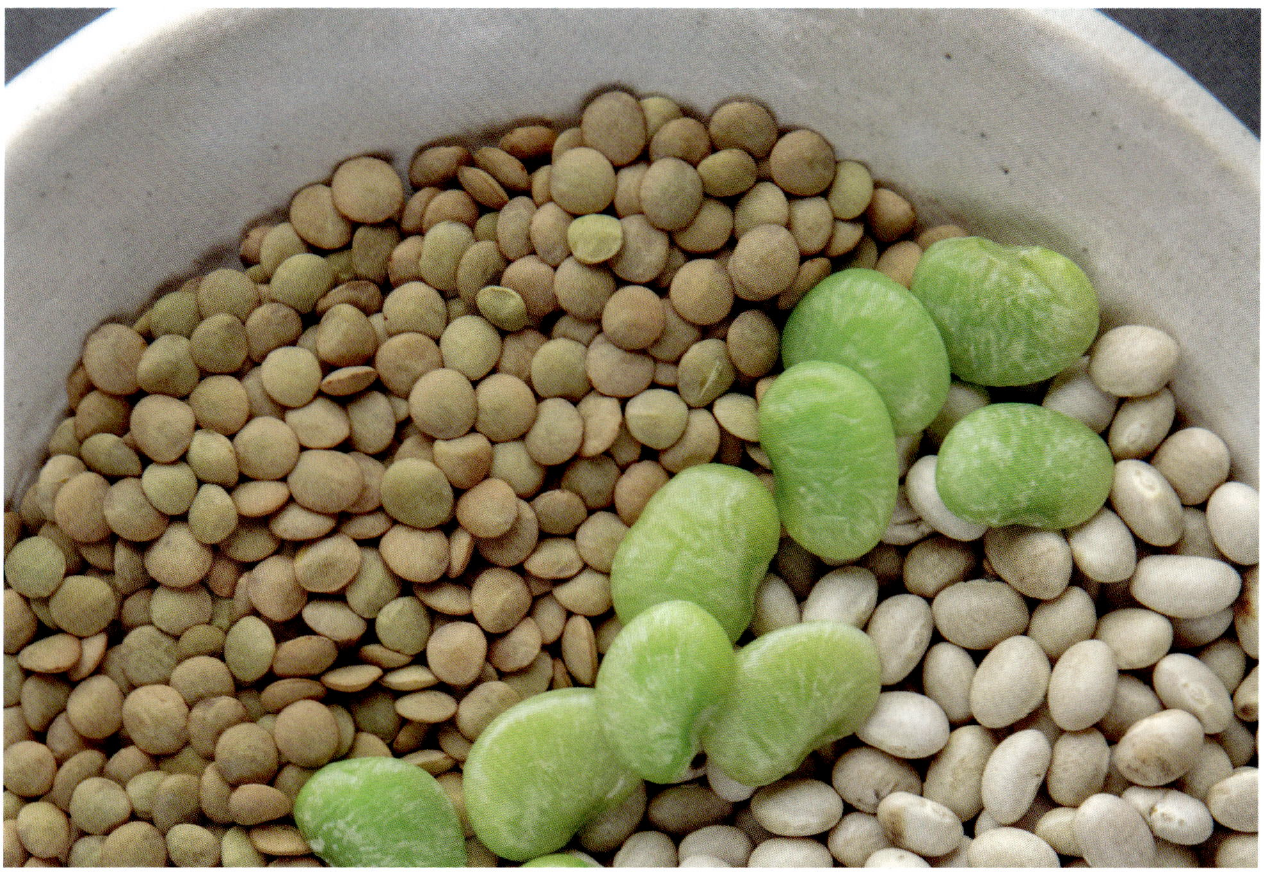

Intro Diet

- White navy beans
- Peanuts

Full GAPS Diet

- White navy beans and peanuts
- Lentils
- Lima beans

Green beans, or haricot verts, are allowed on both the Intro and the Full GAPS diet because they are vegetables. (When eaten together, the bean and the pod of a legume are considered a vegetable.)

> **What is a legume, anyway?** The term "legume" includes beans, lentils, peas (as in split peas), and peanuts, which are of the Leguminosae family. All legumes pose their own challenges to the digestive system, so they must be predigested before cooking or eating.

Intro Diet: White Navy Beans

Using white navy beans is a good option for those who cannot handle nuts and seeds, but in order to render them easily digestible, you must treat them with the three-step process outlined in chapter 9, and it takes about a week or more.

Three-step process for treating white navy beans:

1. Soak or sprout
2. Ferment
3. Cook

Beans also have special complex sugars called oligosaccharides that can wreak havoc on the digestive system. The sugars feed pathogenic and opportunistic bacteria, are very hard to break down, and can cause extreme gastric distress, including bloating and cramping from intestinal gas.

We all know beans can cause flatulence, but this is a sign that your body is having a hard time breaking down your food. If you apply all of the predigestion techniques to beans and legumes before you eat them and you still experience gastric distress such as flatulence, your body is not yet ready to tolerate them. Wait two weeks or more before introducing a small amount again.

> Please note, the only beans allowed on the Intro are white navy beans, not white kidney beans, cannellini beans, or any other white bean.

Intro Diet: Peanuts

As mentioned, peanuts, like white navy beans, are allowed on the Intro diet, but they also need to be treated to make them digestible. You may sprout peanuts as you would nuts and seeds, but the method for soaking them is slightly different. To neutralize the antinutrients in peanuts by soaking, you need to treat them as legumes and soak them in acidulated water—that is, water made acid by the addition of lemon juice, apple cider vinegar, or whey.

If you have concerns about peanuts and aflatoxins, keep in mind that aflatoxins are a family of fungi commonly found in soil. They only become a problem under specific conditions that unbalance the soil, such as poor agricultural methods, drought, and flooding. Not to worry! According to the National Peanut Board, peanut farmers in the United States can rely on safeguards against aflatoxin. And preparing peanuts and any contaminated grain or bean with traditional cooking techniques (soaking, sprouting, and/or fermenting) significantly reduces aflatoxin. So soak! Sprout! Ferment! And then make your own peanut butter.

> **What about peanut butter?** The vast majority of "raw" peanut butter is not really raw—it is a highly processed food. Whether or not they claim to be organic or natural on the label, commercial brands of peanut butter, such as Skippy or Jiff, are made with peanuts that are either deshelled and roasted, or blanched, skinned, sorted, and pulverized. Obviously, both methods of commercial harvesting cook the peanuts. The good news is that these days you can find at least a few brands of raw nut and seed butters (such as VivaPura) that are hand harvested and ground at low temperatures to retain live enzymes.

Full GAPS Diet: Lentils and Lima Beans

On the Full GAPS diet, you may add lentils and lima beans—but they are seeds, and therefore contain antinutrients that must be neutralized by soaking or sprouting, and then cooking. (The method for sprouting is the same as it is for nuts and seeds.)

Just like with nuts and seeds, some techniques predigest beans and legumes more than others. I always suggest doing everything possible to predigest them before you add them to your diet. To do this, you have two ways to go:

Two ways to treat lentils and lima beans:

1. Sprout or soak, then cook.
2. Sprout or soak, ferment, then cook.

You can start with just one process before cooking (such as soaking), and see if it is enough to make the beans tolerable. If not enough, you can always add the other techniques.

Scale of Digestibility: Lentils and Lima Beans on Full GAPS

Hardest to digest →			***Easiest to digest***
Soak, then cook *(soak in acidulated or alkalized water)*	Sprout, then cook	Ferment, then cook	Soak or sprout, ferment, and then cook

Acidulated or Alkalized Water?

Beans and legumes have their own unique soaking requirements for predigestion, including temperature and pH. Some legumes require acidulated water for soaking, while others require alkalized water. To acidulate or alkalize your water, you will add different things (neutralizers) to the water.

> **What is acidulated water?** It is water to which you add an acidic substance. In the case of beans, that could be lemon juice, a mild vinegar such as apple cider vinegar, or whey from yogurt, kefir, or raw milk.

The shape of the bean determines if the water should be acid or alkaline. Kidney-shape beans need alkalized water. Other shapes, round or circular, require acidulated water. (The one exception is black turtle beans, but as these are not on the GAPS diet, we do not need to worry about them.)

White navy beans and lima beans: Alkalized water (water with a pinch of baking soda, not commercial alkaline water)

> **A note on baking soda:** Only pure bicarbonate of soda is allowed for baking on the Full GAPS diet. However, you may use a pinch of baking soda when you are soaking white navy beans on the Intro diet.

Lentils: Acidulated water (water with lemon juice, apple cider vinegar, or whey).

Beans and legumes, if not used quite as often as nuts and seeds, can still play an important role for some in GAPS. The key is to keep in mind that just like with nuts and seeds you must still neutralize their antinutrients in order to continue healing.

Seeds (Nuts, Seeds, Beans, and Grains)

What About Coconut?

8

Coconut. Is it a nut? Is it a seed? Is it a fruit? Where does it fit on the GAPS diet?

Botanically, coconut is classified as a fruit. However, the FDA classifies it as a tree nut, even though most people with allergies to tree nuts do not react to coconut. Coconut has a place on various stages of the GAPS diet, beginning as coconut oil in Stage 1 and progressing to coconut, coconut milk, coconut cream, coconut butter, and coconut flour in later stages.

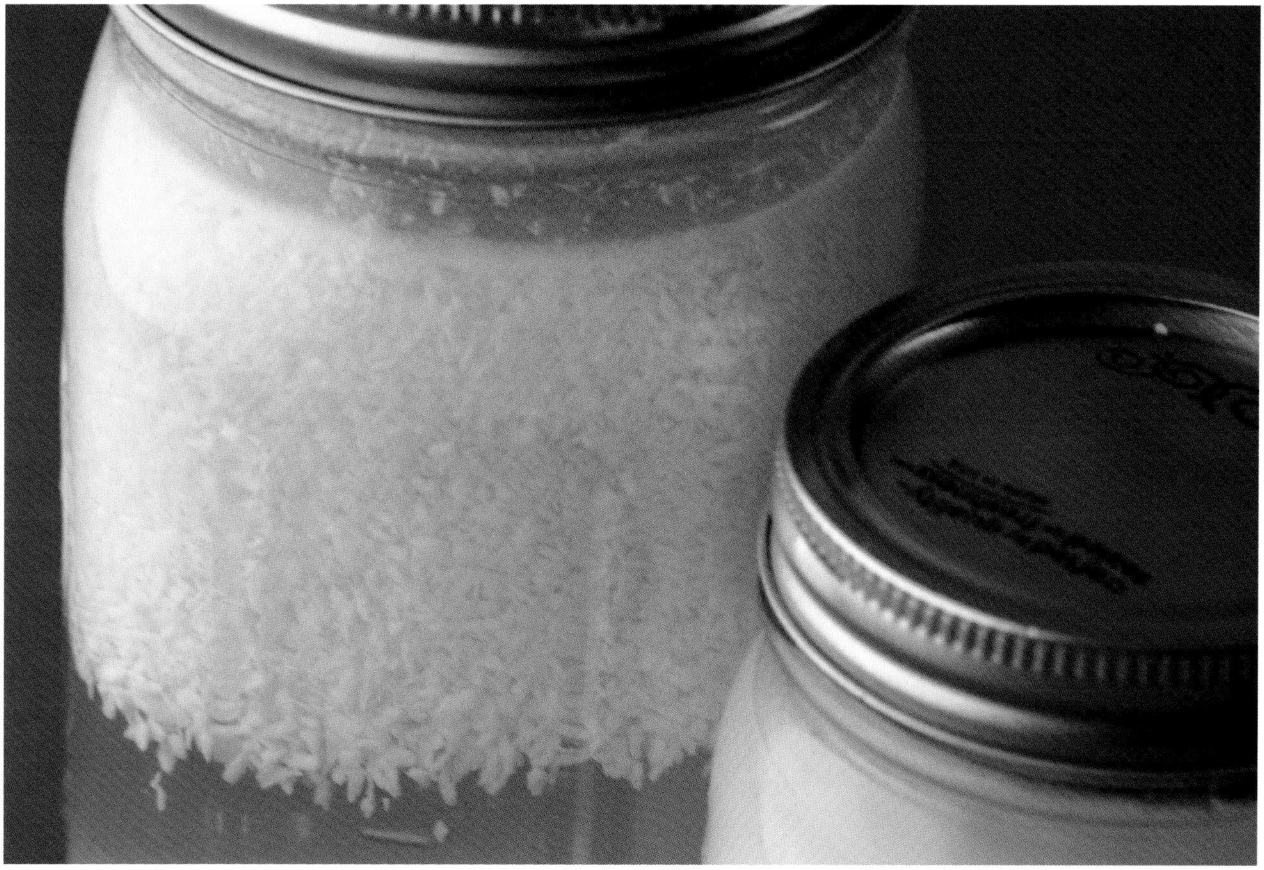

Please note, however, that store-bought coconut flour does not belong on the GAPS diet. It is too high in fiber. You eliminate fiber from your diet on the Intro and only gradually reintroduce it (in the form of the cellulose from raw vegetables) beginning in Stage 5. Store-bought coconut flour has so much fiber that it is never on GAPS—including the Intro and the Full diet. Just imagine rubbing sandpaper on an open wound—ouch! That's what commercial coconut flour does to your gut.

If you would like to use coconut flour, you should always make it yourself. While homemade does not act the same as store-bought coconut flour in recipes, it is easy to prepare and much better for you. Finer and silkier, it contains more moisture than its commercially made counterpart. For recipes, simply experiment and adjust as necessary.

Easy Coconut Milk, Two Ways

Coconut milk: Here's where the fun begins! One way to get at the coconut milk is to use a hammer and flat-head screwdriver. Make a hole in two of the three "eyes" of the coconut. Pour the coconut milk out of one hole. (The other hole helps build up the pressure, making it easier to pour out the milk.) If you like, you can strain the milk through a fine mesh sieve lined with cheesecloth. Pour into a bowl or use a canning funnel to pour into a jar. Once you have poured out the coconut milk, you can split the coconut in half to access the coconut meat.

If you don't want to use a hammer and a screwdriver to break open the coconut, try one of these two easy methods instead.

Easy Coconut Milk I

Ingredients

1 cup organic, unsweetened, shredded coconut
1 cup water

Instructions

1. Place shredded coconut and water in a saucepan. Stir to combine.
2. Bring to a boil. Remove from heat and cool.
3. Pour into a blender and blend thoroughly. Strain through a nut bag, cheesecloth or a linen napkin or towel. (Keep the pulp to make your own coconut flour following the technique below.)

Easy Coconut Milk II

Ingredients

1 cup organic, unsweetened, shredded coconut
4 cups water

Instructions

1. Mix coconut and water, then soak for 4 hours.
2. Blend in a food processor.
3. Strain through a nut bag, cheesecloth, or a linen napkin or towel. (Keep the pulp to make your own coconut flour following the technique below.)

Coconut Flour

Homemade coconut flour is silky and delicious. You make it by drying out the coconut meat, or using the pulp leftover from the coconut milk above. Spread the pulp on a cookie sheet. Place in a 200°F oven or in a dehydrator. When completely dry, which takes about 15–20 minutes or so, pulverize it in a food processor and use as coconut flour in baking.

It bears repeating: homemade coconut flour acts differently in recipes than commercial coconut flour. Homemade has much more moisture and is less fibrous than store-bought.

Another easy-peasy option for homemade coconut flour: You may also make coconut flour by placing store-bought shredded, unsweetened coconut—organic, of course—in your food processor and pulsing it to the consistency of flour. Use immediately, or store in a tightly covered jar in a cool, dark place (cupboard, pantry, or refrigerator) for the longest shelf life.

> Remember, commercially produced coconut flour is not on the GAPS diet. It is like sandpaper on an open wound—your gut!

Coconut Meat

The flesh of the coconut should be white and smell fresh. After you peel it or cut it out of the shell, you may either store it in a container and refrigerate for later use or dry it out in a dehydrator or oven. Use shredded coconut flakes or flour (or a blend) to make coconut butter. If the color of the meat is compromised (yellowish or gray), throw the whole thing out!

Store-Bought Work-Arounds for Coconut

There are times when it is more convenient to purchase store-bought coconut products instead of making them from scratch. And, of course, you can only purchase some coconut products, such as coconut oil and coconut cream, from a store.

The best quality coconut oil is organic and expeller or cold-pressed. It is available refined or unrefined, but the latter is always best as it is less processed. However, unrefined still tastes like coconut. Depending on the recipe, you may not want this.

Refined coconut oil, on the other hand, is nearly flavorless. Liquid coconut oil, sometimes labeled "MCT oil," is the most refined. The medium-chain triglycerides have been isolated from the coconut oil, which is what makes it liquid. This highly refined oil can cause digestive upset (cramps and diarrhea) if you use too much, and too much can be as little as one teaspoon when you first use it.

> Coconut oil is antimicrobial and high in immune-boosting lauric acid. Lauric acid converts to monolaurin, which is a potent antiviral, antibacterial, and antifungal substance. Because of this, Dr. Natasha Campbell-McBride suggests that individuals on GAPS eat coconut regularly.

When purchasing coconut milk or coconut cream, refrain from brands that list guar gum or locust bean gum on the label. Guar gum comes from guar beans or seeds. Locust bean gum (aka "carob bean gum") comes from the seeds of the carob tree. Both are polysaccharides, or starches, which are not allowed on the GAPS diet. Not only is guar gum a starch, but according to the *Journal of Food Science and Technology* (Mudgil et al. March 2014), it is also "a novel agrochemical processed from endosperm of cluster bean… largely used in the form of guar gum powder as an additive in food, pharmaceuticals, paper, textile, explosive, oil well drilling and cosmetics industry."

As usual, it is best to purchase organic coconut milk or cream to avoid the toxins commonly used in conventional growing practices.

Seeds (Nuts, Seeds, Beans, and Grains)
The Techniques

9

Now, at last, the basic techniques of soaking, sprouting, and fermenting! By learning how to apply these time-honored methods to nuts, seeds, and beans, you are unlocking their nutritional power and greatly expanding your GAPS cooking repertoire. Here they are, in a "nutshell."

Keep in mind that you will need whey for the fermenting techniques in this chapter. Store-bought whey powder, however, is a highly processed product and is not permitted on the GAPS diet. Homemade whey prepared from yogurt, kefir, or raw milk is best

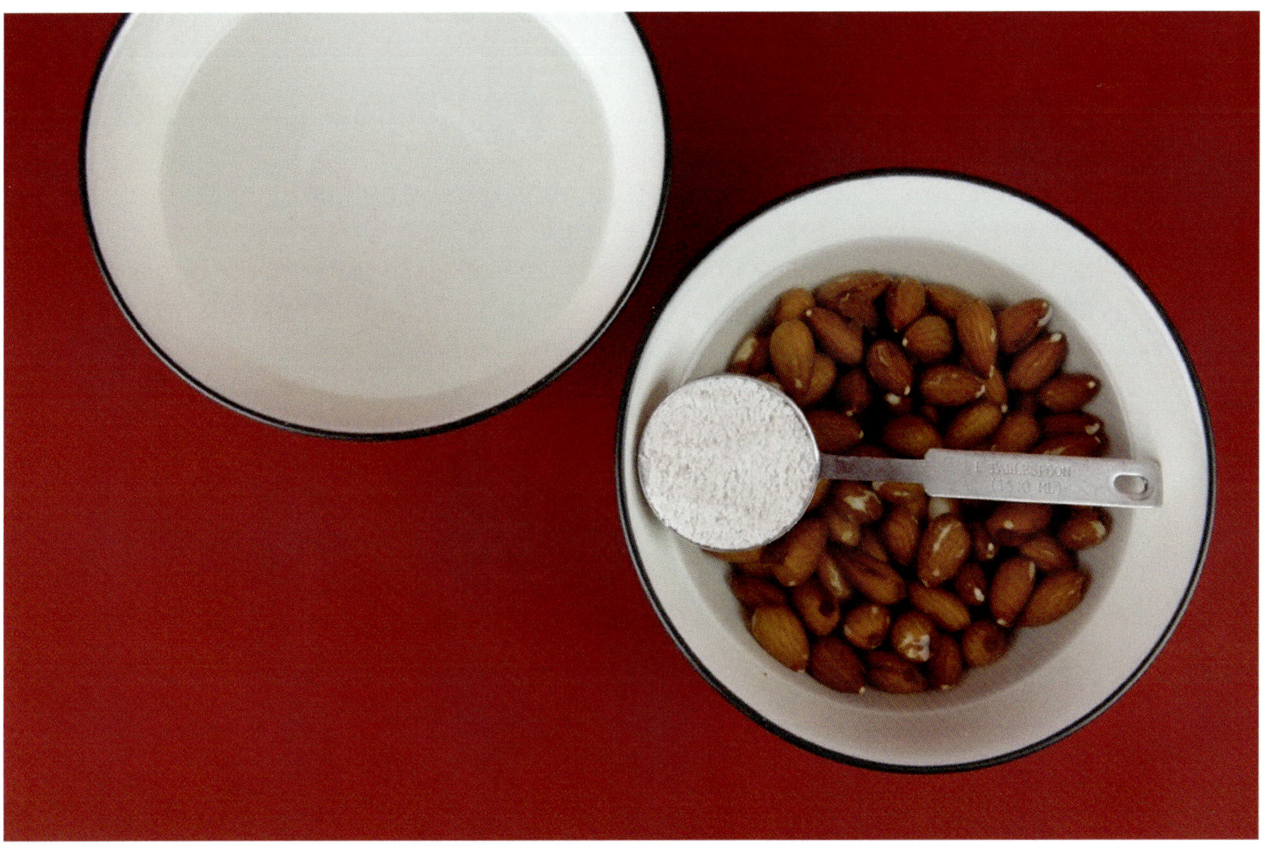

for this healing protocol. And it is very easy to do. The best option for obtaining whey is to get it from cultured dairy products you make yourself—just see the recipes in Section VIII: Culturing Dairy.

If you cannot make your own yogurt or kefir, you may use store-bought cultured dairy products instead—but make sure they are organic, whole milk products from grass-fed or pastured cows, with no fillers such as pectin or guar gum mentioned. But first, it is a good idea to equip yourself with some useful tools that will help you soak, sprout, and ferment nuts and seeds with ease.

Handy Kitchen Utensils and Equipment

- Wide-mouth quart jars with 2-piece lids
- Cheesecloth, lint-free tea towels, or nut bags
- Canning funnel
- Quart capacity (or larger) thermos that will hold hot for 24 hours (this will be noted on label), yogurt maker, or dehydrator
- 2-cup liquid measure, glass preferred
- Fine mesh strainer to fit in 2-cup liquid measure
- Full set of measuring spoons
- Large stainless steel, ceramic, or glass bowl, with plate to fit on top
- Food processor with S blade
- Spatulas or scrapers
- Stainless steel cookie sheets, if possible (if nonstick or another material, line with parchment paper)
- Parchment paper
- Scissors
- Dehydrator (not required but wonderful to have)
- Glass loaf pans
- Muffin tins and paper liners
- 8-inch round cake pans

Soaking Nuts and Seeds

Remember, all you really need to soak nuts and seeds is warm water, good salt, and time.

Ingredients

4 cups raw nuts or seeds (about a pound or so)
Warm water
1 tablespoon good-quality sea salt

Instructions

1. Place nuts or seeds in a large bowl and cover by 2 or more inches with warm water. Add sea salt to bowl and stir.
2. Cover bowl with a plate or towel and set on the counter for 7–24 hours. (Exception: The maximum soak time for cashews is 6 hours. For all other nuts and seeds, 18 hours is required to remove the maximum amount of phytic acid.) After soaking, drain. If desired, you may remove the salt by rinsing.
3. To dry, spread out on a parchment-lined sheet pan and place in the oven or in a dehydrator. Follow guidelines for each option below.

Options for Drying Soaked Nuts and Seeds

If using oven: Set at the lowest temperature possible. This may be the "warm" setting on your oven. (A gas oven with a pilot light is the best option as the light alone is enough to dry nuts and seeds without destroying their enzymes.) Keep in oven for 12–24 hours, depending on the size of the nut or seed and the length of time they were soaked.

If using dehydrator: Turn to lowest setting. Drying at less than 118°F helps retain the live enzymes. However, if you are going to grind soaked or sprouted nuts into flour for baking, do not waste your time preserving their enzymes as baking kills the enzymes anyway.

Soaking Beans and Legumes

Here are general guidelines for soaking beans and legumes. See the handy Soaking Chart below for specifics on the bean or legume you will be using. When it comes to soaking, remember: the longer you soak, the shorter you cook—so soak long!

Ingredients

Lentils, peanuts, lima beans, or white navy beans
Neutralizer
Simmered water

Instructions

1. Bring water to a simmer first (do not use cold water). You will need enough simmered water to cover beans or legumes by at least 2 inches when soaking.
2. Add neutralizer according to Soaking Chart below. (You must make the soaking water either acid or base, depending upon the shape of the bean.)
3. Select soak time according to chart. Change water frequently to keep it hot (adding the neutralizer each time). Rinse at least one to three times during the soaking period.

Soaking Chart for Beans and Legumes

Legume	**Neutralizer** (per cup of beans or legumes)	**Soak Time**	**Replace Water & Neutralizer**	**Cook Time** (lowest heat)
Lentils	1 tablespoon whey, lemon juice, or vinegar	7-12 hours	Up to 1 time *(depending on soak time)*	45-60 minutes *(stir to keep from sticking or burning)*
Peanuts	1 tablespoon whey, lemon juice, or vinegar	12-24 hours	1-2 times	1-2 hours
Lima beans	One pinch baking powder	18-24 hours	1-2 times	1-2 hours
White navy beans	One pinch baking powder	18-24 hours	1-2 times	1-2 hours

Sprouting Nuts, Seeds, and Beans

See the chart on the following page for specifics on sprouting various nuts, seeds, and beans. You may also use this technique to sprout certain gluten-free grains on the Transition diet. (Remember, there are no grains on the Intro or Full GAPS diet.)

Ingredients

Nuts, seeds, lentils, lima beans, or white navy beans
Filtered water

Special equipment:
Glass jar (wide-mouth works best)
Mesh or cheesecloth

Instructions

1. Place about 2 inches of nuts, seeds, or beans in a wide-mouth glass jar. Place a square of mesh or cheesecloth over the jar and secure with ring from lid or a rubber band.

2. Rehydrate by covering with a generous amount of filtered water and letting it sit 12 hours or overnight. Drain and rinse with fresh water.

3. Invert jar and place in a bowl that will keep the jar on a diagonal (see photograph on page 179 for example of jar placement). This will encourage drainage and discourage mold. Place on windowsill.

4. Rinse 2–3 times each day with fresh water until you see sprouts. Nut and seed sprouts will be very small and usually sprout within 2 days. (Note, if sunflower seeds turn black, throw them out.)

Sprouting Chart for Nuts, Seeds, Beans, and Legumes

Type of legume, nut, or seed	Times to rinse per day	Approximate sprouting time	Length of sprout	Notes
White navy beans and lima beans	3 or more	3 days	¼ inch or more	
Lentils	2-3	1-2 days	¼ inch or more	
Almonds	2 or more	2-3 days	¼ inch or less	Sprout will look like a small white dot at tip of nut
Sesame seeds	4	2-3 days	Very small	
Sunflower seeds	2	12 hours or more	Very small	Rinse often to keep from turning black
Pumpkin seeds	2 or more	12 hours	¼ inch	

Notes: Split peas are not included in this chart as they do not sprout. If sunflower seeds turn black, throw them out.

Fermenting Nuts and Seeds

Ingredients

4 cups raw nuts or seeds (about a pound or so)
Warm water
½ cup whey from yogurt, kefir, or raw milk

Instructions

1. Place nuts or seeds in a large bowl. Add warm water to cover by about 2 inches. Add whey. Cover loosely with a plate or kitchen towel.
2. Leave on the counter at room temperature for 24 hours or longer. Drain. Rinse if desired.

Fermented nut and seed flour: You may grind the fermented nuts or seeds into flour and use for the baking recipes in the next chapter. In fact, using fermented flour in baking is the best option. But if you would like to eat them as is, dry them by spreading them out on a parchment-lined sheet pan and placing them in a 200°F oven or in a dehydrator. (But please note there is no need to dehydrate the fermented or soaked nuts or seeds before grinding for baking.)

Fermenting peanuts: Soak or sprout peanuts as above. Drain. Cover with warm water and ½-cup whey and leave to ferment for 5–7 days. Cook in fresh water.

Three-Step Process for Treating White Navy Beans

If you cannot tolerate nuts and seeds, you may use white navy beans instead. But first you must treat them with the following three-stage process:

1. *Soak or sprout:* Soak dry white navy beans 12–24 hours (longer is better) in warm water with a pinch of pure baking soda, changing the water out with just-simmered water when it cools, and adding another pinch of baking soda. Drain and rinse. Alternatively, sprout white navy beans as you would nuts.
2. *Ferment:* After soaking or sprouting, cover with water and ½ cup whey or kefir (per quart of water). Leave to ferment 4–5 days in a warm place.
3. *Cook:* Next, cook in fresh water until tender, then drain. Mash and use in recipes.

Seeds (Nuts, Seeds, Beans, and Grains)

The Recipes

10

You may use all types of nuts or seeds in the following recipes, after applying one or more of the predigestion techniques explained in the last chapter. Keep in mind that fermented nuts or seeds are best for you (most easily digested), followed by sprouted or soaked. Raw nuts or seeds are not good, and roasted nuts or seeds are not recommended. And remember, if you do not tolerate

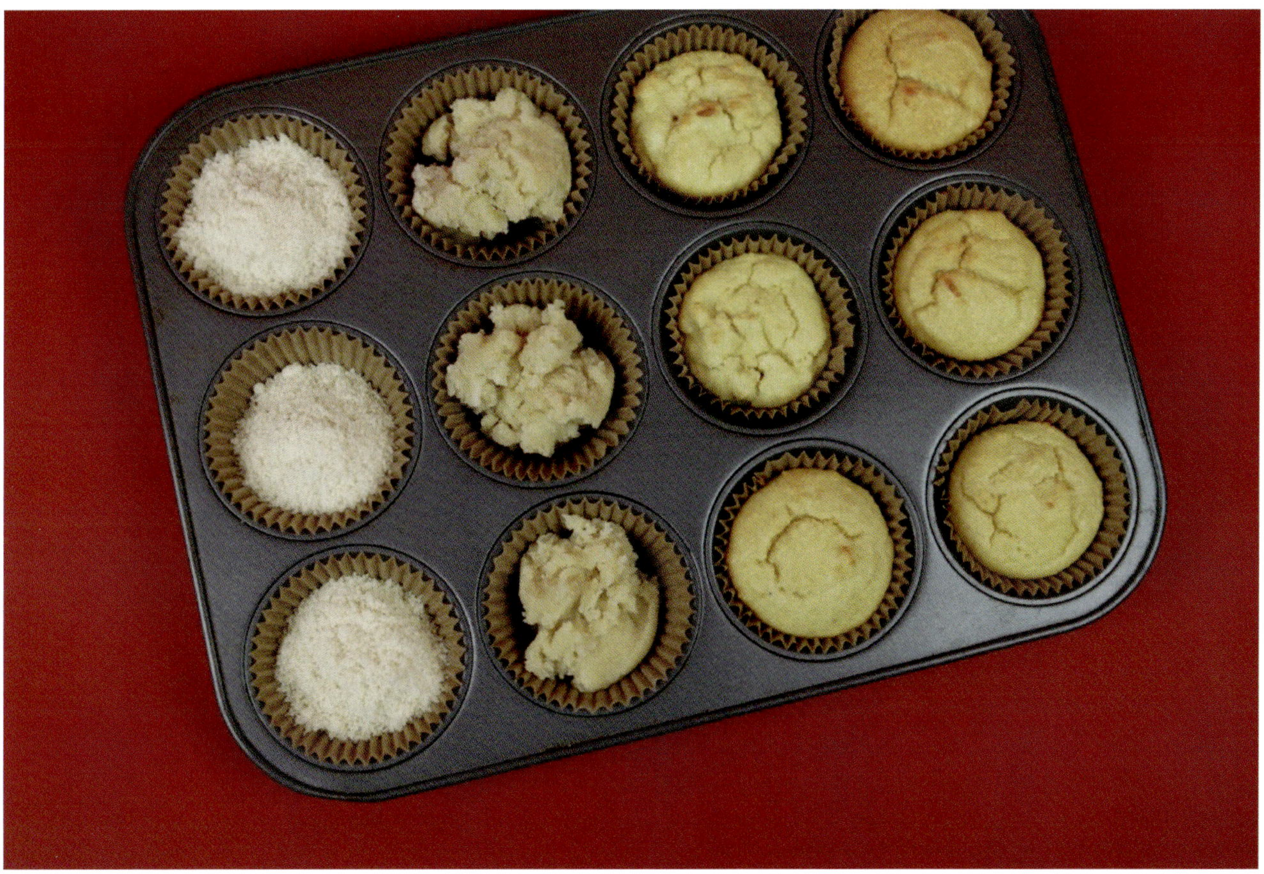

nuts or seeds in any way, you may substitute flour from fermented white navy beans in any of the recipes below, in the same proportions as the nuts and seeds.

A reminder before you get started: Always try to use organic nuts or seeds, which are never irradiated.

Best: fermented nuts or seeds
Good: sprouted or soaked nuts or seeds
Not good: raw nuts or seeds
Not recommended: roasted nuts or seeds

Nut or Seed Butter

If you like, you may add organic, expeller or cold-pressed raw coconut oil to help achieve the consistency you prefer.

Ingredients

2 cups organic nuts or seeds, fermented, soaked, or sprouted
Organic, expeller or cold-pressed raw coconut oil (optional)

Instructions

1. Place nuts or seeds in a food processor with an S blade. Pulse until a butter-like consistency is achieved.
2. Store in a wide-mouth glass jar, tightly covered, in a cool, dark place, or in your refrigerator.

Nut or Seed Butter Pancakes

For these pancakes, you may use more or less nut butter or eggs to achieve the desired consistency.

Ingredients

1 cup cooked and mashed squash, such as butternut or acorn (zucchini can also work if you seed it prior to mashing)
2 or more tablespoons homemade nut or seed butter (recipe above)
3 eggs, organic, pastured, or at least non-GMO
Sea salt, as desired
Grass-fed butter, ghee, coconut oil, lard, tallow, or duck fat (plus butter for serving)

Instructions

1. Mix squash and nut or seed butter together well in a large bowl.
2. Whisk eggs lightly in a small bowl. Add to squash-butter mixture and combine until a batter consistency is achieved. Add sea salt, if desired.
3. Melt your fat of choice in a skillet over medium-high heat.
4. Add tablespoons of batter to pan. Sauté until cooked on one side, then flip and cook on the other side. Serve with butter, ghee, or other desired fat.

Fermented Nut or Seed Flour

Fermented nut flour is the best option for the baking recipes that follow. It is not only the most easily digested, but it also produces very light and fluffy baked goods. Makes about 2½ cups.

Ingredients

2½ cups nut or seed flour (store-bought or homemade)
¼–½ cup whey (Section VIII), yogurt, kefir, or a combination

Instructions

1. Place nut or seed flour in a medium-sized bowl.
2. Add ¼ cup of the whey, yogurt, or kefir and mix well. If necessary, add up to ¼ cup more to achieve a cookie dough consistency.
3. Cover with a plate or plastic wrap. Let sit at room temperature (68–72°F) for 24 hours or more.

Nut or Seed Flour Pancakes

Makes 6–12, depending on size of pancakes.

Ingredients

1 cup nut or seed flour (fermented is best)
1 teaspoon sea salt
4 eggs, organic, pastured, or at least non-GMO
Grass-fed butter, ghee, coconut oil, lard, tallow, or duck fat (plus butter for serving)

Instructions

1. Place nut or seed flour and salt in a large bowl. Stir to combine.
2. In a small bowl, whisk eggs lightly. Add to the flour mixture. Stir well to achieve a batter consistency, using more or less nut butter or eggs, as desired.
3. Melt fat of your choice in large sauté pan over medium heat.
4. Add spoonfuls of batter to pan. Sauté until cooked on one side, then flip and cook on the other side. Serve with butter, ghee, or other desired fat.

Variation for Pancake Crisps: Heat leftover pancakes in a low to medium oven until crisp. Delicious. And crispy!

> **No nonstick pans, please!** As always in the GAPS diet, you want to minimize the toxins entering your body. Glass or cast iron is preferred. However, if you only have nonstick baking pans, be sure to line them with parchment paper.

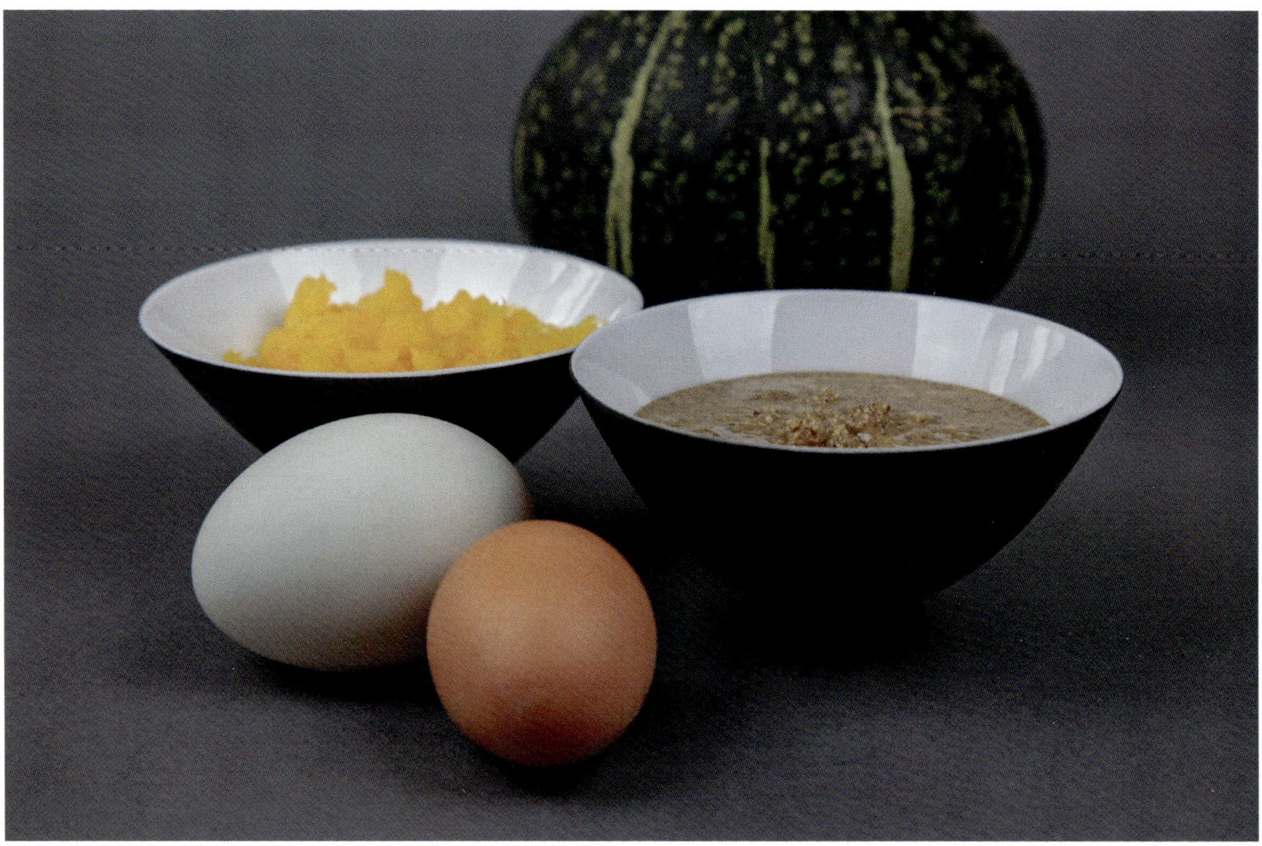

Basic Bread or Muffins

Using the fermented nut or seed flour recipe from page 201 is the best option here. The amount you need depends on if you use soaked, sprouted, or fermented nut or seed flour or a store-bought version. Makes 1 round pan (8–9 inch), 1 loaf pan, or 1 dozen muffins.

Ingredients

3–4 eggs, organic, pastured, or at least non-GMO
¼ cup yogurt (best), or melted butter, coconut oil, duck fat, goose fat, lard, crème fraîche, or kefir
About 2½ cups nut or seed flour (fermented is best)

Instructions

1. Preheat oven to 350°F. Line pan with parchment paper (or muffin pan with cupcake liners), greased with a healthy fat.

2. Beat eggs in a medium bowl. Add one of the fats or dairy products listed above. Slowly add flour. The batter should have the consistency of porridge. Use an additional egg to achieve porridge consistency, if necessary.

3. Bake in center of oven: 15–20 minutes (for muffins) or 45–60 minutes (for loaf or cake pan). Cook time depends on consistency of batter, size of your pan, and heat of your oven. To test for doneness, insert a clean, dry knife in the center of the loaf. When it comes out dry, the bread or muffins are done. (Test muffins at 10–15 minutes and loaf or cake pan at 45 minutes.)

Variations on the Basic Bread Recipe

In addition to choosing a loaf, cake, or muffins, you can also be creative with the following variations to the basic recipe. Once you can tolerate the following ingredients, try adding 1–1½ cups to each batch you make. As always on a healing diet, it is best to use organic ingredients whenever possible.

Variations for the Intro diet:
High-quality sea salt
Fresh herbs
Tomato paste or puree
Fresh or frozen berries (thawed and drained) or chunks of apple
Grated carrot
Chunks of peeled, seeded pumpkin
1 avocado, well mashed

Variations for the Full GAPS diet:
All of the above, plus:
Chopped nuts or seeds
Dried herbs
Dried fruit (dates, raisins, apricots, figs, or other fruit of your choosing)
2 ripe bananas, well mashed (include an additional egg)
Cheese (such as Parmesan, aged cheddar, or other hard cheese)
Cinnamon or other spices

Pizza

This pizza is allowed on the Full GAPS diet. The Basic Bread recipe is called for here, preferably a batch made with fermented nut or seed flour. If you cannot tolerate cheese, you may use homemade mayonnaise instead.

Ingredients

1 batch Basic Bread
Organic tomato puree
Sea salt
½–1 cup of any of the following: sliced bell pepper (any color), mushrooms, cooked meat or sausages, tomato slices, chopped greens, anchovies, fish, prawns, or pineapple, in any combination
1 cup grated cheddar or Parmesan cheese, or homemade mayonnaise

Instructions

1. Preheat oven to 300°F. Line a baking tray with greased parchment paper. Spread out the Basic Bread dough like a pizza crust (about ¾-inch thick).
2. Bake 30 minutes. Check with a knife to see if it is cooked through. Let cool.
3. Spread tomato puree and a dash of salt over the crust. Add toppings as desired and cover with grated cheese or mayonnaise. Eat as is, or pop back into the oven for 3–5 minutes, until cheese is melted. (Do not heat if using mayonnaise.)

Pizza Muffins

This recipe makes about 12 muffins and is allowed on the Full GAPS diet. For the Basic Bread, it is best to use a batch made from fermented nut or seed flour.

Ingredients

One batch Basic Bread
Organic tomato puree or paste
1 teaspoon each dried basil and dried oregano
Sea salt
1 cup grated cheddar or Parmesan cheese (if tolerated)

Instructions

1. Preheat oven to 300°F. Mix all ingredients together well. (You may reserve some of the cheese and tomato puree or paste for the top of each muffin.)

2. Spoon batter in muffin tins lined with parchment paper liners.

3. Bake about 15 minutes. Check center of muffins with a toothpick to see if they are cooked through. Let cool. Enjoy!

Nut or Seed Milk

Makes about a quart. If you like, you can retain the nut or seed meal for baking. If you cannot purchase organic nuts or seeds, make sure they are not irradiated. It would be best, of course, if you soaked, sprouted, or fermented the nuts or seeds first.

Ingredients

1 cup organic nuts or seeds, organic if possible
2–3 cups of pure water to blend, plus more for soaking

Instructions

1. Soak nuts or seeds in warm water for 12–24 hours. Drain.

2. Blend in a food processor with 2–3 cups pure water. Mix well.

3. Strain through a nut bag or fine mesh sieve lined with cheesecloth. The liquid is nut or seed milk! (Retain nut or seed meal for baking if desired.)

Seeds (Nuts, Seeds, Beans, and Grains)

Frequently Asked Questions

11

Does the temperature of the water matter when soaking nuts, seeds, or beans?

Warm water is beneficial for soaking nuts, seeds, and grains. But for beans, it is an absolute requirement. You need warm water to get the beans to soften and open. The hotter the water, the faster they open and predigest. Simmered water works best.

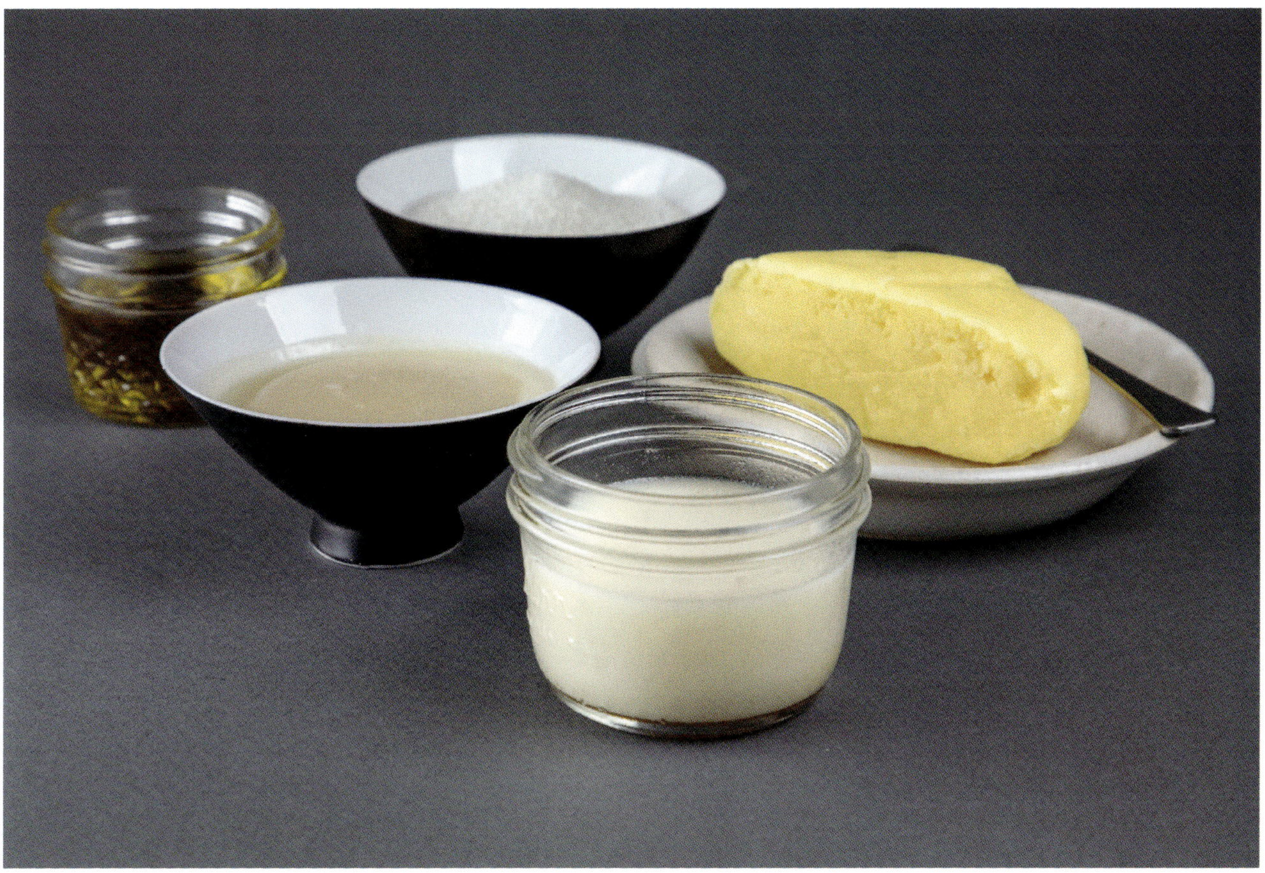

What is simmered water?

I often receive questions about the "simmered water" on my Preparing Whole Grains and Legumes chart. This is water kept right below the point of boiling (about 212°F).

What should I do if my seeds mold when I sprout them?

If you see black mold (or any other color) on your sprouted nuts or seeds, throw them out!

Why do I need to change the soaking water for beans? How often do I need to do it?

As I mention above, beans open or soften in hot water. In cold water they will not open at all, and they may even contract. Therefore, I suggest changing the water every time it cools to room temperature (and adding a new neutralizer at the same time). Don't go crazy, though. If you change water once every 8–12 hours, it will be enough.

What is a healthy fat?

Dr. Natasha Campbell-McBride is very clear that saturated animal fats are optimal for human health and healing. As such, they're a large part of the GAPS diet, and you should use them liberally. Traditional animal fats are safe for cooking and baking because they don't change their structure when heated. Healthy, traditional fats include beef, bison, or lamb tallow, lard from pigs, schmaltz from chickens, and duck or goose fat. But these fats are healing only if they come from pastured animals. You are whatever you eat eats. Toxins are stored in fats, so you do not want fats from animals given GMO feed, antibiotics, or growth hormones. Fats should come from healthy, grass-fed animals only.

What about fats from the vegetable kingdom? Coconut oil is a healthy saturated fat with the added benefit of being antimicrobial (see chapter 8). Virgin and cold-pressed or expeller-pressed olive oil is also healthy, but you should never heat it, and you should not use it in baking recipes for nuts or seeds. (Olive oil is not included until Stage 4 of the Intro diet.)

What about salt?

Many people are concerned that salt is not good for them. However, most people on the GAPS diet have mineral deficiencies, so for them salt is essential. Choose a salt that lists the amount of trace minerals on the package. I suggest any with a minimum of 50 trace minerals or more, and with no fillers or anticaking agents. Sea salt is usually the best.

What about canned beans?

Forget the canned beans. Soaking your own beans is less expensive and more sustainable. Not to mention the fact that it makes the nutrients more available to you. Though canning may neutralize a small amount of phytic acid, it also exposes the beans to very high temperature and pressure, denaturing the protein and other nutrients in the beans.

Can I use my pressure cooker to cook beans?

Forget the pressure cooker. The very high temperature and pressure denatures the protein and other nutrients in the beans.

What about nut or seed oils?

Nut and seed oils play a very important role in the GAPS diet as a supplement. Make sure they are unrefined and unadulterated. Always use them cold (never heat). Dr. Natasha recommends using oil blends that contain more omega-3 than omega-6. A good nut or seed oil will have a 2:1 ratio of omega-3 to omega-6. Some of these may contain evening primrose oil or flax seed oil as a base. Hemp oil and straight flax oil (flax seed supplements) are not recommended as the former is too heavy on omega-6 fatty acids and the latter is too heavy on omega-3 fatty acids.

Seeds (Nuts, Seeds, Beans, and Grains)

Bonus Chapter! Working with Grains on the Transition Diet

12

What is the Transition diet? Exactly what it sounds like: the diet you eat as you gradually transition to foods not allowed on GAPS. You will know you are ready to transition off GAPS when all of your digestive symptoms are gone.

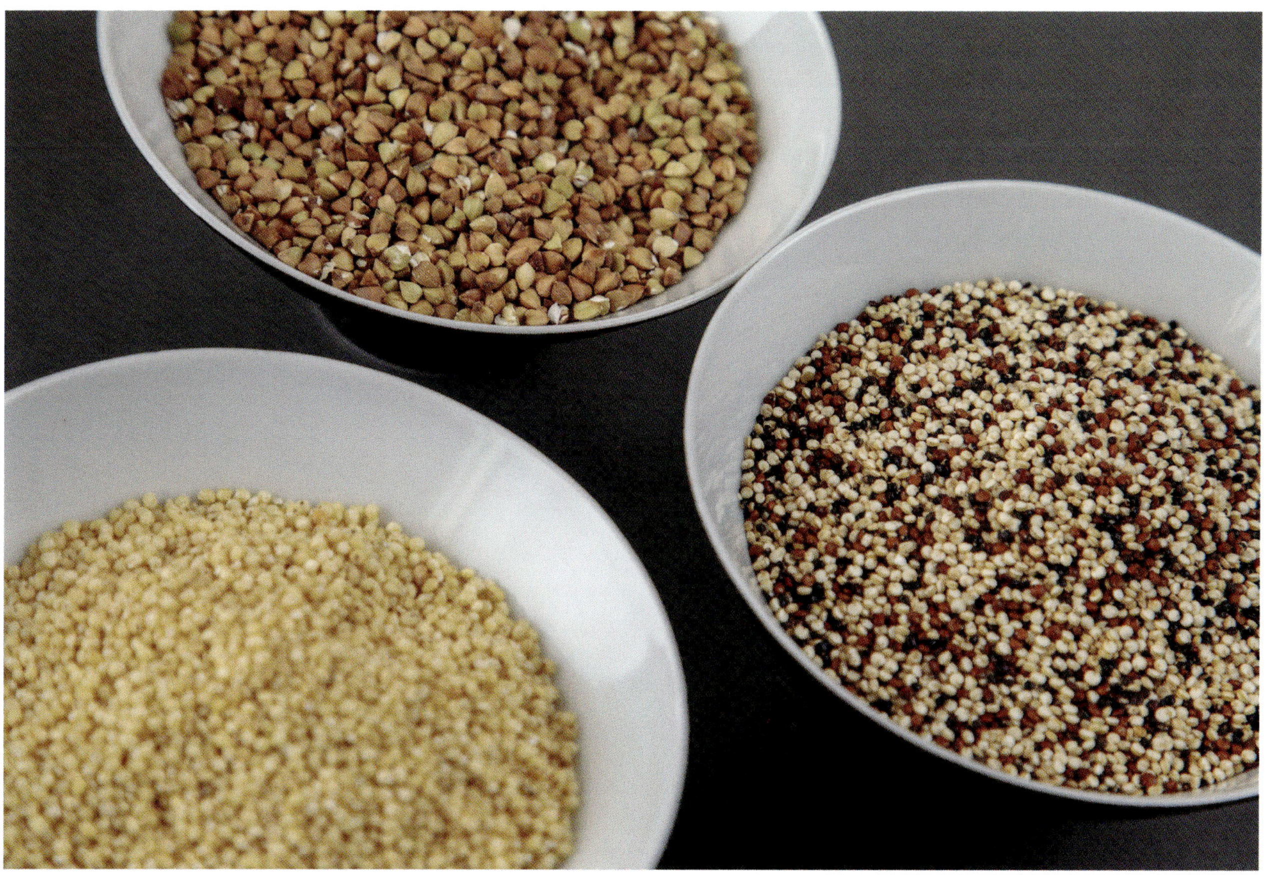

> Rather than transition, some people feel best staying on a GAPS-style throughout their lives. This is perfectly okay. Listen to your body, and don't rush yourself to transition off GAPS.

When you no longer experience digestive distress from any of the foods on the diet, you are finished with Full GAPS. For most people, this takes about two years. Once you transition off, you gradually introduce grains back into your diet. As I mentioned previously, *grains are also seeds*. And of all of the seeds, grains are the hardest to digest.

That is why it is so important to learn how to introduce grains into your diet. You want to make sure they will not cause you any digestive distress. As you know very well by now, when you introduce a new food on GAPS, you introduce just a little bit of it, slowly, watching for any signs of intolerance, be they physical, emotional, or mental.

The first grains you introduce back into your diet are gluten-free, specifically buckwheat, millet, and quinoa, and you must ferment them first. Begin with 1–2 tablespoons per day, and be sure to eat them with plenty of good, healthy fat (grass-fed butter, ghee, olive oil, coconut oil, or any other natural animal fat). Fats slow down the digestion process and help control spikes in blood sugar. Grass-fed butter also assists with neutralizing any phytic acid in the grain—so go ahead and slather it on!

Fermenting Buckwheat, Millet, or Quinoa

Make sure the water is warm, not hot. You don't want to kill the lactobacilli!

Ingredients

1 cup grain, rinsed
½ cup whey (see Section VIII)

Instructions

1. Cover grains with warm water by 2 inches. Add whey and cover loosely.
2. Leave at room temperature to ferment (buckwheat 2–3 days; millet 4–5 days, quinoa 1–2 days). After fermentation, drain and rinse. Then cook.

You may introduce the fermented grain back into your diet by cooking it in Meat Stock or water with good salt, serving with meats and vegetables, or using it in place of flour for baking (see Sourdough Pancakes recipe below).

After you successfully introduce fermented grains into your diet, try sprouted or soaked grains. However, fermentation is the best predigestion technique, so these other methods will be more challenging to your system. Again, start with 1–2 tablespoons and eat with a healthy fat. Watch for symptoms of digestive distress. If you experience any, stop eating the grain for two weeks or more before reintroducing it back into your diet.

Sourdough Pancakes

According to Dr. Natasha, these sourdough pancakes are a great first way to introduce grains back into your diet once you can tolerate them.

Ingredients

1 cup organic buckwheat or millet flour, or a combination, freshly ground if possible
1 cup organic, whole-milk kefir (homemade is best)
3 eggs, organic, pastured, or at least non-GMO
2 tablespoons or more pastured butter, ghee, or other healthy fat, for sautéing
Sea salt, as desired

Instructions

1. Mix flour and kefir well in a large bowl. Cover loosely with a plate or towel. (The bacteria and yeast in kefir like oxygen, so don't make it airtight.)

2. Leave at room temperature 24–36 hours.

3. Whisk eggs lightly in a small bowl. Add to flour mixture and stir to combine until it reaches the consistency of batter.

4. Melt butter, ghee, or other healthy fat in pan over medium heat. Add batter and sauté pancakes until cooked.

Section XI | What to Eat After GAPS: The "Well" Diet of Weston A. Price and Nourishing Traditions

When people ask me what they should eat after the GAPS diet, my answer is the "Well" diet. This diet is based on the way of eating advocated by the Weston A. Price Foundation (WAPF) and laid out in Sally Fallon's influential cookbook *Nourishing Traditions*. (More recently, it has also come to be known as the Wise Traditions diet.)

Before I go on, let me offer a little background: In the 1930s and 40s, Dr. Weston A. Price traveled around the world to study traditional peoples, their diets, and their health. He later documented this research in his book *Nutrition and Physical Degeneration*. Sally Fallon's *Nourishing Traditions* is based in large part on Dr. Price's work.

GAPS itself is a therapeutic diet designed to heal and seal the gut and, in turn, the symptoms caused by an impaired gut. Once you have healed and sealed your gut through GAPS and transitioned some foods back into your diet, you are ready to cook and eat in a way that will help you keep and maintain your wellness. Thus, I call it the "Well" diet.

What is the Well (or Wise Traditions) diet? Put simply, it is the best-quality food you can find, prepared with traditional *Cooking Techniques* that both predigest the food for you and preserve and enhance the nutrients in the food. These are the very same techniques that you have been using all along on the GAPS diet! Preparing nourishing stocks and broths. Culturing dairy products. Lacto-fermenting vegetables, fruits, and tonics. Soaking, sprouting, and fermenting nuts and seeds. And finally, on the Transition diet, using all of these techniques to expand your culinary repertoire to include grains and beans.

According to the Weston A. Price Foundation (WAPF), the foundational principles of the optimal human diet are as follows:

- Nutrient-dense whole foods (no processed food)
- Fat-soluble activators (vitamins A, D, and K2)
- Healthy fats: 30–80% of diet (26–76% saturated and monounsaturated fat; nearly equal amounts omega-3 and omega-6 fatty acids)
- Animal foods in every diet
- Organ meats
- Lacto-fermented vegetables, fruits, meats, and condiments
- Soaked and sprouted seeds, nuts, and beans
- Soaked, sprouted, or fermented grains
- Cultured dairy
- Raw and high-enzyme foods (including raw milk and raw meat)
- Gelatin-rich bone broths

Start with the highest quality ingredients: Food should be fresh, local, sustainably raised, organic or biodynamic. Meats from animals raised on pasture (grass-fed). Eggs from hens raised on pasture, eating bugs and grass. Traditional fats such as lard, tallow, pastured butter, animal fats, coconut oil, and olive oil. Certified raw dairy (from pastured cows), not pasteurized (subjected to heat) or homogenized.

Stephanie Selene Anderson's *Put Your Money Where your Mouth Is! Guide to Healthy Food Shopping* is an excellent source for not only learning more about these foods but also where to find them.

Prepare these ingredients in a way that maximizes their nutrition: Eat some of your food raw (or cooked less than 118°F) to preserve the nutrients and enzymes. Add high-quality fats to vegetables and meats so you can absorb the fat-soluble vitamins and other nutrients more easily. Use predigestion techniques that unlock nutrients in food and allow your body to easily absorb them. Ferment some of your foods and eat ferments with every meal. Soak, ferment, or sprout all beans, legumes, pulses and grains prior to cooking. And eat cultured dairy products.

As you can see, these techniques should already be familiar to you from following the GAPS diet. And when you transition off the diet, you will start eating grains and a greater variety of beans, legumes, and pulses. It is likely that you will never go back to eating bad, processed food again. Or at least not for long. The price is too high.

Foundational Principles of the Optimal Human Diet

Characteristic of Optimal Human Diet	Why These Foods	Where These Foods Are Found	Avoid
Nutrient-dense whole foods	Full spectrum of nutrients available	Biodynamic and organic foods Sustainably grown and raised foods Foods grown or raised close to their source Fresh produce Foods that are not processed in a factory	Foods with labels Foods processed in a plant or factory Foods made of "food fractions" Refined sugar High-fructose corn syrup White flour Canned foods Refined or hydrogenated vegetable oils Skim or low-fat milk Milk powders Protein powders Toxic additives and colorings GMOs
Fat-soluble activators: Vitamins A, D, and K (*K2 only found in animal foods*)	Required for mineral absorption	Fish livers Shellfish Organ meats, especially liver Pastured butter from cows eating fast-growing grass in the spring and fall Cod liver oil	Earth Balance Fake butter of any kind Margarine Trans fats

Foundational Principles of the Optimal Human Diet

Characteristic of Optimal Human Diet	Why These Foods	Where These Foods Are Found	Avoid
Healthy fats *(30–80% of diet; 26–76% saturated and monounsaturated fats)*	Required for the absorption of calcium and other minerals Build immunity by fighting microbes in the gut Lower levels of LpA in the blood (LpA causes clotting and atherosclerosis) Prevent compromised brain chemistry (60% of brain is composed of fat) Required by cells to function properly and maintain their integrity (50% of every cell membrane is made up of saturated fat) Protect the liver from toxins (including alcohol) Provide energy to the heart in times of stress Required by the lungs (fatty acids in lung surfactant normally 100% saturated)	Polyunsaturated oils naturally occurring in grains, legumes, nuts, fish, animal fats and vegetables (4%) Saturated fats from animals (tallow, lard), coconut and palm oil (26-76%) Monounsaturated (olive oil)	Earth Balance Fake butter of any kind Margarine Trans fats

Foundational Principles of the Optimal Human Diet

Characteristic of Optimal Human Diet	Why These Foods	Where These Foods Are Found	Avoid
Animal foods	Protein, protein, protein! Animal proteins more easily absorbed and utilized by the body than plant proteins	Fish and shellfish (wild-caught only) Land and sea mammals (pasture raised and wild) Eggs Milk and milk products Reptiles Insects Whole animal consumed: muscle meat, organs, bones and fat (organ meats and fat preferred)	Farmed seafood Commercial meat from concentrated animal feeding operations (CAFOs)
Organ meats	Super foods! High in easily absorbed vitamin A	Beef, bison, chicken, lamb, turkey, etc.	
Lacto-fermented vegetables, fruits, and beverages	Predigestion Ease of digestion Ease of nutrient absorption Increased enzymes Increased vitamins, including vitamin C Probiotics: lactic acid producing bacteria Increased immune function	Fermented pickles, sauerkraut, etc. Fermented beverages Fermented preserves and chutneys Almost anything can be fermented!	Pasteurized fruits, vegetables, and beverages
Soaked and sprouted seeds, beans, legumes, pulses	Neutralizes antinutrients that block nutrient absorption (phytic acid and enzyme inhibitors) Predigests long-chain carbohydrates	Your own soaked seeds, beans, legumes, and pulses Some commercially available sprouted seeds, beans, legumes and pulses	Canned beans, legumes, and pulses

Foundational Principles of the Optimal Human Diet

Characteristic of Optimal Human Diet	Why These Foods	Where These Foods Are Found	Avoid
Soaked (fermented) and sprouted grains	Neutralizes antinutrients that block nutrient absorption (phytic acid and enzyme inhibitors) Predigests long-chain protein molecules (gluten)	Your own soaked (fermented) grains Sourdough Commercially available sprouted grains and sprouted grain breads	Commercial prepared breads, crackers, muffins, etc. that are not sourdough or sprouted
Cultured dairy (milk and cream)	Predigests lactose and casein Increases enzymes and vitamins Ease of nutrient absorption	Cultured Butter Full-fat, organic, plain yogurt Cultured cream, crème fraîche Full-fat, organic kefir	All UHT (ultra-high-temperature-processed) dairy All commercial dairy Homogenized dairy (when possible)
Raw foods and high-enzyme foods	Contribute to digestion of other foods Full of vitamins and enzymes	Raw milk Raw meat Raw vegetables	

A Note from the Author

I hope that you have enjoyed reading *The Complete Cooking Techniques for the GAPS™ Diet* and that you will use it often. I wrote the four books in my original *Cooking Techniques* series with the goal of taking the mystery out of the Gut and Psychology Syndrome nutritional protocol and teaching readers how to cook for the GAPS diet with ease. In gathering this trove of information together, I soon realized that I would need to set the series within the context of the full GAPS journey: the Intro diet, the Full GAPS diet, and the Transition diet. Now, with this complete volume, I am confident that you possess all of the tools and confidence you need to start healing. I have truly enjoyed shedding some light on the GAP Syndrome and the GAPS diet. It has been a labor of love, and I am optimistic that it will serve you well for a long time to come. These are timeless, traditional techniques that you can use as part of a healthy, real-food diet long after you are "off GAPS." Wishing you all the best on your journey back to well-being, and always!

My best,
Monica

About the Author

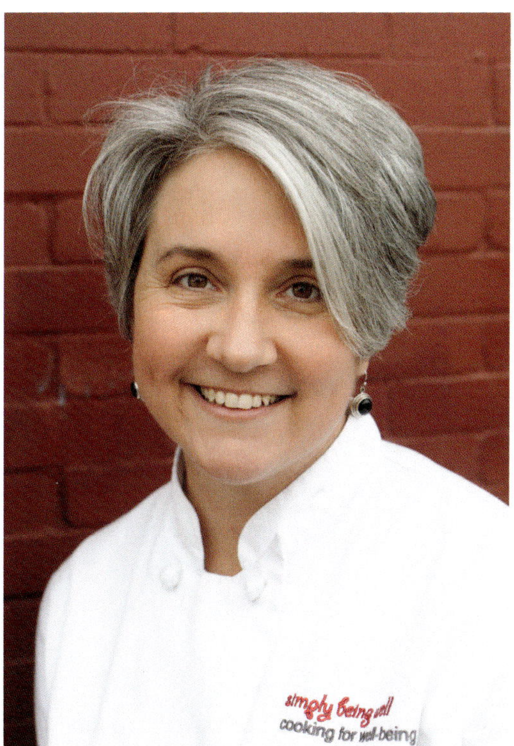

Monica Corrado, MA, is a teaching chef, a holistic Certified Nutrition Consultant, and a Certified GAPS Practitioner. Since 2018, Monica has been part of the GAPS Practitioner Training team with Dr. Natasha Campbell-McBride. A dynamic speaker, consultant, and author, she is passionate about illuminating the connection between food and well-being. Monica lives to give others the tools they need to cook nourishing, traditional food as well as the knowledge and inspiration they need to educate others. Monica has been teaching food as medicine for more than thirteen years, after eighteen years in sustainable food sourcing and preparation, menu design, and management. From 2000 to 2005, Monica owned and operated The Basic Feast, one of the only organic catering companies in the Washington, DC, metro area offering nourishing food from local, organic, sustainable farms. Monica has been a leading activist in the sustainable and local food revolution for over almost twenty years. In 1998, she became a founding member of one of the first CSAs in the Washington, DC, metro area and was invited to be a member of the Honorary Board of the Weston A. Price Foundation.

Monica has spoken on public television on the issue of children and nutrition, and she took part in the White House Chefs Move to Schools initiative. She has appeared in numerous newspaper articles, and in September 2010 she was on the front page of the *Washington Post* Food Section for an article on her fermentation classes titled "Fermentation: A Wild Way to Make Food Come to Life!" In Monica's private practice, she works with her clients to clear up the causes of any symptoms or dis-ease in the body. Monica's current efforts focus on the brain-gut connection and overall gut health. Her desire to help people thrive and come to balance through food led her to develop groundbreaking cooking classes on the GAPS healing protocol years ago. Much of her work is centered around helping those with any issue connected to gut health, including ADD, ADHD, Asperger's, autism spectrum disorders, autoimmune disorders, and allergies. Monica also works with cancer survivors, and she addresses fertility issues and "failure to thrive" diagnoses. She helps people who feel "stuck" or cannot seem to find relief from symptoms. Through her intuitive insight, she often finds the crucial missing piece that will help her clients continue their journey to well-being.

In her effort to reach people globally, Monica offers cooking classes both online and around the world that focus on traditional food based on Weston A. Price and the Gut and Psychology Syndrome diet. She has also started her own Cooking for Well-Being Teacher Training program, which passes on the skills of traditional food cooking and how to teach this skill to others. Graduates of her Traditional Foods Teachers program have taken Monica's teachings to Canada, Mexico, Hong Kong, and throughout the United States.

For more information about Monica, visit SimplyBeingWell.com.

About Dr. Natasha Campbell-McBride

Dr. Natasha Campbell-McBride is well-known for developing the concept of GAPS (Gut and Psychology Syndrome), which she details in her book *Gut and Psychology Syndrome: Natural Treatment for Autism, Dyspraxia, ADD, Dyslexia, ADHD, Depression, and Schizophrenia*. Thousands of people around the world follow the highly successful GAPS nutritional protocol to help themselves and their families.

Note: Gut and Psychology Syndrome™ is the trademark and copyright of Dr. Natasha Campbell-McBride. The right of Dr. Natasha Campbell-McBride to be identified as the author of this work has been asserted by her in accordance with the Copyright, Patent, and Designs Act 1988.

Resources

The following books, articles, and online resources will go a long way toward helping you not only continue your GAPS journey but also maintain your health for decades to come.

Find SRP on Social Media

- Like Selene River Press on Facebook
- Follow Selene River Press on Twitter and Pinterest

Find Simply Being Well on Social Media

- Like Simply Being Well on Facebook
- Follow Simply Being Well on Twitter

Books to Bridge the GAPS

The Art of Fermentation by Sandor Ellix Katz

Breaking the Vicious Cycle: Intestinal Health through Diet by Elaine Gottschall

Excitotoxins: The Taste That Kills by Russell Blaylock

GAPS Stories: Personal Accounts of Improvement and Recovery through the GAPS Nutritional Protocol compiled by Medinform Publishing

Gelatin in Nutrition and Medicine by Nathan Ralph Gotthoffer

Gut and Psychology Syndrome: Natural Treatment for Autism, Dyspraxia, ADD, Dyslexia, ADHD, Depression, and Schizophrenia by Dr. Natasha Campbell-McBride, MD

Healthy 4 Life: Dietary Guidelines from the Weston A. Price Foundation

Nourishing Broth: An Old-Fashioned Remedy for the Modern World by Sally Fallon Morrell and Kaayla T. Daniel

Nourishing Traditions: The Cookbook That Challenges Politically Correct Nutrition and the Diet Dictocrats by Sally Fallon Morrel, with Mary G. Enig, PhD

Preparing Whole Grains & Legumes (chart) by Monica Corrado. This beautifully illustrated laminated chart is perfect to hang in your kitchen.

Put Your Money Where Your Mouth Is! Guide to Healthy Food Shopping by Stephanie Selene Anderson

Real Food Fermentation, Preserving Whole Fresh Food with Live Cultures in Your Home Kitchen by Alex Lewin

Weston A. Price Foundation Shopping Guide: This handy pamphlet lists specific brands and contact information for many of the highest quality foods on the market. This same information is also available in the Find Real Food app from the Weston A. Price Foundation.

Wild Fermentation by Sandor Ellix Katz

Articles

Three online articles that outline the beauty of meat stock and bone broth—and the importance of understanding when and how to use them on the GAPS Diet.

"The Dark Side of Bone Broth" by Monica Corrado (SeleneRiverPress.com)

"Why Broth Is Beautiful: Essential Roles for Proline, Glycine and Gelatin" by Kaayla Daniel (WestonAPrice.org)

"Stock vs. Broth: Are You Confused?" by Kim Schuette, Biodynamic Wellness (TheHealthyHomeEconomist.com)

Essential Websites

Continue your education and deepen your knowledge with the following online resources.

SimplyBeingWell.com: Monica's website offers a deep well of knowledge about the connection between real food and well-being.

RealMilk.com: Learn more about the Campaign for Real Milk, launched by Sally Fallon and the Weston A. Price Foundation to promote universal access to clean raw milk from pasture-fed cows.

WestonAPrice.org: The Weston A. Price Foundation is your source for a wealth of accurate information on the Wise Traditions Diet and so much more. Here you'll also find the Wise Traditions journal, edited by Sally Fallon and the Wise Traditions Podcast.

AvivaRomm.com: Aviva Romm, MD, bridges traditional wisdom with modern medicine. Her website is full of information on women's and children's health, online courses, and book recommendations to help you support your lifestyle changes.

Price-Pottenger.org: Information on nutrition and health, organic and nutrient dense food, recipes and food preparation, fertility and prenatal health, food allergies, natural medicine, and so much more.

Online Resources for the GAPS Diet and Certified GAPS Practitioners

Have a question about GAPS? You will find the answer at these websites.

Doctor-Natasha.com: Dr. Natasha Campbell-McBride's website is an incredible resource for GAPS families and for Certified GAPS Practitioners alike.

Gaps.me: Also from Dr. Natasha Campbell-McBride, this is the original Gut and Psychology Syndrome™ website. Featuring original GAPS recipes and information on the Full GAPS diet, supplements, fussy eaters, and so much more. Also includes an important searchable FAQ where you can find answers from Dr. Natasha on a range of questions regarding all phases of the GAPS nutritional protocol. From locating a GAPS practitioner to learning how to sign up for practitioner training courses, this is a valuable online resource.

GapsDiet.com: Collects all the latest updates and news related to GAPS. You will also find a portal for GAPS resources and support.

SCDiet.net: Find information about the Specific Carbohydrate Diet, the foundation of the GAPS diet. A great resource for food, the SCD mailing list, and SCD-friendly practitioners.

BreakingtheViciousCycle.info: Another great source of information about the Specific Carbohydrate Diet, which has helped thousands of people with various forms of bowel disease and other ailments vastly improve their quality of life.

PecanBread.com: Here you'll find the most comprehensive list for foods allowed on the SCD, as well as strategies for success, free advice, and links to important articles.